I0449642

SOUL WINDOWS
SECRETS FROM THE DIVINE

SUSAN Z RICH

Copyright 2012 Susan Z Rich,
All rights reserved.

Published by eBookIt.com

ISBN: 9781456609856

No part of this book may be reproduced in any form or by any electronic or mechanical means including information storage and retrieval systems, without permission in writing from the author. The only exception is by a reviewer, who may quote short excerpts in a review.

TABLE OF CONTENTS

INTRODUCTION

As a seasoned intuitive, emotional addiction counselor, author, motivational speaker, workshop facilitator and holistic therapist of twenty years, I have listened to most versions of life's challenges in one form or another. The one question that repeatedly came up was, "Why is this happening to me in my life now"? I asked the same question about my own life challenges many times. One of them being my own personal health challenge of Stage Four Breast cancer 15 years ago in which I chose to heal myself naturally without chemotherapy or surgery. Through a systematic and guided process of staying energetically observant to the similarities of life cycles everyone went through, I was able to see a pattern of divine communication. These communications sent from the divine inner self to assist the soul living out its scripted life journey. Those communications are in the form of scheduled life cycle signals to prompt change and growth. When these spiritual coding signals are activated, it opens a Soul Window. A Soul Window is similar to a memo sent to the dreaming soul to have a look at what point in this life adventure will change begin to happen. Meaning, what did you come here to do, accomplish, release or possibly finish and is it now time?

As baby boomers are hitting the most challenging Soul Window of Chiron Return (the 50-year birth cycle) and the young generation is experiencing instantaneous karma, all old paradigms of beliefs and foundations are crumbling. Soul Windows allow you to make a connection with your inner Divine self, get a spiritual pep talk and a new game plan for the next life cycle of your living incarnation. Something like your divine life coach calling you to the sidelines and giving the next plays on your life journey. Helping you to find your "Muchness" and to let your "God Sparkle" shine! I hope the information I was gifted to share about Soul Windows will help you experience this life journey in more joy and enlighten you with a few "Aha, that makes so much sense" moments.

Namaste
Susan Z Rich
www.szrwhitewings.com

HOW SOUL WINDOWS HELP US REMEMBER OUR LIFE SCRIPT

After 20 years of sharing emotional and intuitive counseling, helping clients to learn how to become empowered, I discovered an amazing life process I call Soul Windows. A perfectly balanced divine communication system to help you on this journey you call life. Soul Windows are the tools of the divine self that shake up all the emotional belief systems you designed for yourself to create a karmic release of separation from Oneness. You will accept a belief and go along with dysfunctional ideas created by tribal, family or environmental conditions and then you hit a certain age and something does not sit well with you anymore. The usual comments depending on what Soul Window we are talking about is "No, I do not want to do that anymore, I am unhappy and do not know why or I just cannot take this anymore." Your personal beliefs attract and create your physical reality. If taught as a child that love always comes with the conditions of being hurt and disappointment, then all your life interactions are based on those beliefs. You would repeatedly create relationships that would support that concept of love because it is all you know. Even though it may bring you hurt and unhappiness time and time again, the comfort level of familiarity and the fear of the unknown keeps you in the loop. Your identity is wrapped completely around that belief system. It is not an authentic truth, but it is your truth and more than likely your family, tribal or even religious truths. Somewhere on your life journey, your divine self will set it up to question your loyalty to those beliefs through the Soul Windows. You are not going to change any dysfunctional belief unless you can convince your sub-conscious (Inner Child emotions) there is something better to replace it.

I used a self-hypnosis program of Empowered Thinking to help accomplish that goal with clients. If the Inner Child begins to hear repeatedly what they believed to be love might actually be something else, they can make a choice of rejecting the old and replacing it with a more loving version. You must first experience a new version of belief that makes you feel better about yourself. Once you experience a feel good moment, the Inner Child will happily embrace the new belief. If it feels good then it must be better, it makes sense on every level. Your sub-conscious is just a big emotional computer program that controls your feelings and responding behavior based on the core beliefs that are running. You can begin to make choices that do not support hurt or abandonment and begin to experience the unconditional love that is truly yours by birthright. Soul Windows are the tools the divine self uses to help the Inner Child learn how to trust that knowing inner voice. They also help the adult listen to the knowing voice of divine reason instead of the ego's screams of fear. After repeatedly giving the subconscious feel good emotional beliefs, the Inner Child's behavior will embrace the new idea and start making choices accordingly. You realize you like how the new ideas make you feel and the change begins. Healing change comes down to whose opinion you value more, someone else's opinion of you given to you as a young child or how you want to feel about yourself now. You must first have a feel good belief program running in your sub-conscious mind before you can make that choice.

After watching clients change to the better with the Empowered Thinking program, I began to notice that every age group had certain life challenges that came about regardless of what their story was. There was a pattern to this madness, as they say. The astonishing fact is that you have in your soul's etheric field, scheduled life cycle signals designed to become active at certain age groups in your life journey. These energetic life cycle signals, created to open particular Soul Windows, bring a change of desires and situations for you to begin a new life chapter. Allowing that program to do what you came here to do, for the soul to experience growth. It is like a window opening in order for the soul to become remapped and rewired to make change. Look at it from this perspective, you are sleeping and dreaming and then the lights turn on briefly, getting your attention and giving you the agenda for the next life cycle, which by the way YOU wrote.

People attached to the good opinion of others have deep self-doubts about where their own value comes from. Co-dependence is a common behavior of low self-esteem and sometimes is so subtle you cannot recognize the real issue. If someone has the capability to push your buttons or make you do something you are not happy doing, then you are attached to their good opinion of you. You need to have that person embrace the same beliefs and opinions you have or you feel challenged over the control you think you are losing. When you finally disconnect yourself from the good opinion of others, you feel a real sense of freedom and a great burden lifted. It can be a

24 hour a day job trying to figure out how to get others to do what you need them to do. Trying to second-guess someone else's thinking and figure out what YOU have to do to get their approval is emotionally exhausting, frustrating and futile. When you finally realize this, you have that incredible epiphany and ah ha moment of healing. You now know your opinion of yourself is the only one that really counts and actually has the most value. There is a spiritual saying that when you shift your perception of disharmony and finally see for the first time the cause of it, you realize you have just missed the <u>obvious</u>! Usually that happens when you finally become aware you were never going to win at being loved unconditionally anyway. Someone was always going to out think or out manipulate you to get their needs met first. Soul Windows assist you with bringing about this new wisdom to help you see things from an authentic perspective. Trying to live a co-dependent life and thinking eventually you will figure out how you are going to get your needs met without having to compromise is the ever elusive gold ring. Depending on someone or something outside of yourself to feel whole, safe, loved or of value is always going to be just out of your reach. It is like holding your breath; sooner or later you will realize there is someone who is one-step

ahead of you in the need department and about to collect it from YOU! No matter how slick you are, how nice you are, how smart you are, how controlling you are or how clever you think you are, you are going to meet your match to force you to grow out of that need. YOU designed it that way! You are finally going to understand the situation is not what you thought it was or they are not doing what you expected them to do. When that happens, all the illusory foundations come out from under you. Then your defense mechanisms will kick into gear: feeling fear, anger, violence, blame, control, withdrawal, manipulation or whatever is your tool of choice. Your other choice is being humble and in gratitude of being shown where NOT to travel. This choice is never one the ego prefers as it forces you to take full responsibility of co-creating your circumstances. When a Soul Window opens, the ego must step back and allow space for change as divine truth will always overrule ego's falsehoods. The ego is never happy about that!

I had many metaphysical and spiritual clients but also some that were not into spirituality but knew there must be some version of a God and some kind of plan, or hoped there was. I even counseled atheists who took the approach of what the heck, I am so miserable what do I have to lose. Especially when I explained the Inner Child does not really care if you call God "Sam", it is the concept of being One and a part of something bigger than they are. They were always relieved to find the counseling program was not all metaphysical woo-woo and full of praise God and Jesus! It just made a lot of sense there had to be something more in the game we were playing called life. Maybe the program should have been called: "Common Sense Spirituality". Considering the over the top mystical approach to healing is what usually keeps people from grasping the concept that in the end, it is all YOU. No angels, no mystical beings, no punishing or rewarding God, (they always like the part of a non-punishing God but are never thrilled with the idea of a God who does not reward for good behavior) no heaven to reach or hell to be afraid of. This life is just your beautiful soul having a wonderful adventure from a script that you wrote. I am not saying angels and all our wonderful light beings are not there to help, they are just all a reflection of you and your beliefs. One of my favorite sayings to get that point across is, "If you wrote the script for your life, then I would guess you can rewrite it". Soul Windows open at important life markers, helping to see you have the power to make changes in your life script. We are spiritual beings having a human experience, not the other way around. This life is not the IT or the only game in town. When we do not understand the game we are playing, it becomes scary in the belief that an unseen someone or something is pulling the strings in your life. When we carry this belief, wanting to embrace rescue me energy always interferes with accepting the responsibility for your own success of so-called failures. To get this point across, the first thing I always told clients is your life is not a crapshoot rolled by God. YOU designed it for a purpose and if you examine the patterns in your life, it will become obvious what that life lesson is. Soul Windows open to remind you by creating continual change in your life circumstances and assist you in accomplishing those life lessons. I was blessed with the intuitive ability to see one's life journey without the ego's smoke and mirrors defense program that fiercely defends an illusion of separateness and aloneness.

People who usually showed up for counseling or the therapy program were in the throws of severe life changes such as extreme fear, a health crisis, abandonment and self-doubt. In the past, they were just at a point of being stuck in life but with the new intense energy on earth now, it seemed everyone was going through volatile changes. No one is having the luxury of extended time anymore. They found the old way of pushing things aside, putting off problems, pretending issues did not exist or hoped they would just go away was not working anymore. The Empowered Thinking program taught them to shift the place of responsibility from out there in someone else's hands as in: It is God's will, in God's hands, it is out of my hands, it is Divine will, there is nothing I can do about it, etc. It put the responsibility where real power begins, with YOU! YOU are that divine will in partnership. YOU are co-creating your life with the divine self and YOU are the one making the decisions on how this life is going to unfold. That is free will. Soul Windows are designed to remind you on your life journey, what free will looks like.

DISCOVERING LIFE CYCLES THROUGH SOUL WINDOWS

After listening to all the different client age groups and their life difficulties, I started having a spiritual awakening myself. I became very disillusioned with reading all the spiritual how to self help books and participating in healing workshops, whether my own or someone else's. The big zinger came when I found myself to be completely bored with my own emotional addiction program. I recognized this particular jumping off place as I had encountered it before when I created the Empowered Thinking program. Once again, I had that feeling of not accomplishing what I wanted with clients and my own journey of self-discovery. Everything I was hearing at this point was sounding something like this: "Blah, blah, blah, blah, blah!" I realized I was filtering the same client phrases over and over again. The difference this time was I became painfully aware I was also saying the same old key words. I was not happy or satisfied after each therapy and counseling session. I began hearing stories from spiritually aware people who seemed to be doing all the right things but had finally come to a place in their lives stuck in a loop of behavior or circumstances that would just not go away. No amount of prayer, counseling, workshops or rituals were making much of a difference. There were stories of 27-year marriages just disintegrating overnight. I was also seeing major health issues unexpectedly coming up everywhere and easygoing clients exploding in anger and frustration. I had to ask myself what the HECK was going on here? The boredom of hearing me saying all the cliché support words like: "you have to find your self-esteem, fill your life with the light and love of Holy Spirit of God or now is the time to start feeling your self-worth, etc. was getting intense! All these wonderful spiritual words, metaphysical sayings and belief foundations I had been using for so many years and very attached to the benefits of them were obviously not working anymore. I started noticing client's eyes glazing over when I used these pat metaphysical phrases. They had heard them all before. It was at that point I became aware that the blah, blah, blah was also coming out of my mouth this time. I was becoming very dissatisfied with the dialogue of the self-empowerment program. The other thing I was fast becoming aware of was an inner dialogue of that divine voice I have always tried listening to. It was chatting me up big time once again.

What this brought about was an emerging pattern I had experienced before. I was now getting introduced to a new format of spiritual communication that I would eventually recognize as Soul Windows. This would take the Empowered Thinking concept to a new level. An emergence of patterns began to emerge with specific life cycle changes and commands, happening at certain ages in the soul's growth and journey. The dilemma was how do I make these new soul markers understandable to clients? I went back to my tried and true method of separating client notes, this time by age instead of emotions and feelings as I did with the Empowered Thinking program. When done, I was startled to see how clearly a pattern of soul commands guiding us through our life's journey. Soul Windows open at selected age groupings, allowing guidance and communication from the divine self. Every age group dealt with the same core issues, each in their own fingerprinted design but still the same emotional issues connected with them.

The Soul Window concept came about when specific life cycle patterns became apparent observing my clients scheduled appointments. I started having clusters of age groups coming for therapy sessions and intuitive counseling. For example, I would get appointments week after week that were in the age group of 20's to 30's. Then for a time, another age group of 40's to 60's, then from 30's to 50's. I am used to being setup by the divine by now, knowing when that enlightened presence is beginning to direct a spiritual change of perception for me. I have always taken the approach the gifts I use in counseling and helping others is also about my own life's journey and growth. The big question was how to use this new information on Soul Window life cycles to help clients understand and use it to empower their own life journey.

Most of the time, all new information makes itself known in my meditations. I do not define meditation as most people do as I meditate in motion. Power walking every morning for three miles is what I call quiet meditation. There are times when I have done the whole three miles and do not remember walking a step but had lots of Aah Hah moments! I would love to say these amazing spiritual breakthroughs come from that 2:30AM spiritual window when you sit straight up in bed and have that incredible clarity. Instead, I have had many of those moments mid stride on my walks. I am very sure the people who have seen me walking this circle for years talking to myself have long gotten used to me stopping and yelling something glorious! I am also used to being labeled a little bizarre in my thinking and how I react to things, so I am completely detached from the good opinion that I am that very nice woman but yes just a little odd.

I am once again on a new spiritual quest! When walking at full speed, I am praying and asking to be shown what I have to know to make sense of all of it. I am now driven and know my divine self is trying to show me a great teaching tool to take my counseling to the next level, but what the hell is it? This is when I usually move into what I call my OCD mode; you know...obsessive, compulsive, disorder! I totally go into that energy when I know spirit is pushing me to awaken to some new truth.

The first piece of information given to me was that I was completely bored with the dialogue used in counseling sessions. I had enough of watching my clients eyes glaze over using all those old worn out spiritual phrases that are textbook healing tools. For example, I started saying your self-confidence or inner strength is your "Muchness". How many times do we say in our day of activities that we would like to have much more of this or much more of that? The concept is; being much more than you believe you are in the moment and believing that you are capable of even bigger boundaries. I would explain being in your Muchness is feeling fearless in the belief of total faith and trust in your own self-confidence and self-empowerment. Faith and trust in your own decisions being guided by the knowing voice from within regardless of how things may appear in the moment. Knowing everything will somehow turn out wonderful for you. You do not need anyone to tell you or try to control a guarantee from God or someone else that is out there for that truth. Of course, teaching clients that concept and having all of them getting it, would put me out of a job! Lol.

What most fearful people do not understand about being fearless, is they believe the fear must completely go away. Then they will be brave enough to say, do or have what they would like. Fear is not that bad of a thing, as it is a very powerful tool used by your divine self to bring about change. The bottom line reality of having Muchness is what I call experiencing the moment of spitting in the devil's eye (another name for one's arrogant, manipulating and taunting ego). You know you have the fear but you finally come into what is the first transition of the healing phase, Righteous Anger. You have had enough! That is when you make the announcement to yourself and the universe: "Alright, I know I am afraid but I am going to do it anyway! That is the first stage of healing, finding your Muchness through Righteous Anger or "spitting in the devil's eye". Soul Windows will challenge your fearlessness many times throughout your life journey to help you face this lesson.

It was at this time I also started giving clients a new affirmation called the "Fake It Till You Make It" affirmation. It goes something like this: "Regardless of how things may appear in my life at the moment about (fill in the blanks) and this challenge." "Regardless of how I feel about this life challenge, I know with every fiber of my being and without a doubt this will turn out wonderful for me, somehow, someway." "Why? "Because God and Divine Self have my back and is helping every step of the way." What that affirmation does is keep your emotional Inner Child from painting you into the corner of "IT", meaning if you do not have, get, be or create a certain outcome, the world will come to an end for you or you will DIE! If you think that statement is a little over the top, you must remember you are dealing with a child's feelings of fear that has no gray area of reasoning like an adult. The affirmation helps give your fearful Inner Child hope there is a way out beyond what they can see in that moment. That is the key to containing fearful, out of control behavior and feelings. You have to give strong hope of a better outcome to erase the irrational childlike fears the adult is experiencing.

The second part of the dialogue change I made was explaining what happens after you get your Muchness for the first time. The first stage of this process being Righteous Anger, you get pissed off! Soul Windows will set up many emotionally challenging life circumstances for you in order to push the buttons needed to make you intensely react. The difference now is you are not angry with anyone or anything, nor is there any blame game going on. It is the kind of anger that you slap yourself on the forehead and make the statement, "What the hell was I thinking?" The second stage of the healing process is Introspection, where you start taking a good look at who you really are and the choices you have made in the past. Once you are in your Muchness mode, you now have the tools to be brave enough to look at the good, the bad and the ugly about yourself. The third part of the process is a Metamorphous of your behavior, emotional reactions and responses. This is where I would always tell clients to ask to be filled with the light, God's love, Holy Spirit and pray to find your inner light. Those glazed eyes would happen again! One day on my meditation walk, I looked at one of the pond fountains and as the sun caught the water spray, it just sparkled. It stirred the memory of asking to see the true form of one of my angel guides, Archangel Michael. What I saw was the sparkling light show of a dazzling, iridescent, gel like helix form. I remember being totally blown away by the sheer luminescent properties of what I was seeing but also a little disappointed there was no huge white winged apparition which so many of us associate as being angels. It was at that moment seeing the sparkling fountain that I came up with the definition of the "God Sparkle" within. I started using that phrase to explain being filled with God, divine light or Holy Spirit. I would say to clients when the whining and victim energies would start,"You need to get into your Muchness and get your God Sparkle on, girlfriend!" The reactions I was getting from that statement was, "Oh yeh, I like the way that makes me feel." "I know what you are trying to get me to see now". I started seeing clients making the connection and paving the way for the final stage of healing called the Epiphany. That shift of perception puts you into a new dimension of life and commonly called a miracle of change. The foundation for this is basically, once you see you cannot un-see. The Soul Windows help you open your eyes and experience authentic feelings to assist you in these shifts of perception.

The final dialogue change came from the self-confidence, worthiness and value shift I was looking for. I started using the phrase, "you need to get a "Tude" about who you are and what you are if you are going to get what you want". Of course, the inevitable question would be, "what is a Tude"? I would put my hand on my hip; stick out my chest and say, "attitude, attitude, girlfriend"! " You have to believe YOU ARE ALL THAT and coming to the table with valuable stuff, not always looking and hoping that someone is going to bring you something valuable so you feel good about yourself!" I could see I was now starting to get somewhere with this new approach. I do so apologize to all the male readers in staying in the feminine gender, as I did have many male clients also. Obviously, when I had a male client I changed the approach just a little and put more testosterone into the delivery. What I finally began to see was the emotions and feelings of a new idea getting across to them. This was the new awareness I was looking for, it was ALL based on the feelings you have about yourself. Your childhood situations and the adults that decided your life choices when you were young formed the adult emotions you were now dealing with. Soul Windows open at specific emotional ages to bring about maturity and wisdom. They also start the process to help you un-do any childhood defenses. The agenda was to get you to embrace the feel good emotions about yourself, you would then know the difference between being a victim and being in charge of your life.

The next step to this new Soul Window concept was to catalogue client's counseling sessions by age group. Since I completely embrace the belief that we write the scripts for our life journey and we certainly do not arrive here without assistance, then we must have some kind of handbook we brought along with us. This is what that handbook looks like. We have energetic scheduled life cycle signals that go off within our etheric life field (and no, I am not talking about the so-called alien implanted chips that healers claim to find in their subjects, although anything is possible). These life cycle signals awaken and prompt us to make the necessary changes on our journey to grow and complete what we came here to do. Each one of these scheduled life cycle signals opens a portal I call Soul Windows. This allows the dreaming soul to stir, awaken and bring about the necessary life adjustments for those changes at selected ages. Everyone and I mean everyone goes through these soul changes. A meeting place where the soul looks through a window of change and is directly coached and guided by their Divine higher self. This is of course where free will comes into play. The divine self is always assisting in the creation of these Soul Windows, urging the soul to make change. Whether you choose that option of change is entirely up to you. I like to think of it as divine rah, rah cheerleading for us. The free will given us is always about choices made by the individual soul from either authentic joy or fearful doubt. We all came here to experience and accomplish an agenda to bring about the soul's growth and the awareness of no separation between the soul and the divine intelligence known as God and by many other wonderful names. The point to this journey is to recognize home as within and not separate from the Oneness of All. God is not out there, life is not out there and we should not be looking out there for it. Everything is within and One within us. That is what we are here to sort out and embrace.

Our journey neither begins nor ends with a goal but is completely about the experience. We are here to experience the emotions of everything until the feeling of being separate from the divine within us and separate from each other, are no longer felt by the soul. Whether that takes ten more lifetimes or a thousand, it is irrelevant to the divine self.

The divine within will experience those emotions through us, expanding in awareness as we grow and evolve. In the script we write for ourselves from wherever it is that we go when we are between incarnations, we make our choices on how the journey is going to unfold. This game plan has all the design foundations of what we want to experience. The purpose of that life script is always about the soul finding resolution for a karmic imbalance and releasing it. Depending on how deeply emotionally imprinted the imbalance is, it may take lifetimes. You and only you decide how long and in what way the game is going to play out in your life journey. You pick the players, the storyline and the tools to help you learn what is needed. It is all you, your life is not a crap shoot rolled by some divine being sitting in the heavens saying..."yeh, snake eyes on this guy", "His life is going to be one miserable experience." Just does NOT happen that way.

The players in your life journey are always from your soul family, written in your scripts playing different characters in many lifetimes. They are thrilled to help you and usually the part they play in your life is designed as a learning experience for them too. So do not be so fast to judge a parent, family member, partner or friend for causing you massive pain or harm in your life as everyone agrees to play out their roles for you, just like YOU asked them to. Sometime your worst nemesis is one of your dearest soul family members and is doing a great favor for you. You ask them to make you miserable to get the needed lesson or experience and they say they would be happy to, done deal. It is a dirty job but somebody has to do it for you. Soul Windows also allow you to recognize when a soul family contract is finished, and it is time to move on. Regardless if that soul family member got the lesson or not, you are the one making the choice. Always remember that lifetimes to the soul's divinity is like taking on and off a set of clothes when they become worn and dirty and then putting on a fresh life. No big deal and it is that emotionally detached. The soul's life experience should neither be judged bad nor good; just a part you are playing out at that moment in divine time.

It is this concept clients usually had the hardest time accepting when I told them they chose their parents. Their reactions were either one of two…"I did not!" or "What the hell was I thinking?" But you did and the reason why was for the necessary genetic coding to experience your soul's learning journey. The soul will also choose whether they will have matriarchal or patriarchal mapping, meaning which parent you will genetically bond with to help your experience unfold. You see the effects of a child's genetic imprinted journey of self-discovery with comments of being a momma's boy or daddy's girl. A matriarchal child, will have the mother's genetic heritage traits that soul needs to accomplish what is necessary to do in that lifetime. The reality of parenting is the matriarchal soul child really does not care who in their soul family the father is as long as the required genetics are there. The attachment to the mother is predominant in their feelings for one another. It does not necessarily mean a harmonious agreement but an understanding between them, nonetheless.

The same rules apply to a patriarchal child, the genetics mapped from the father and the soul not placing much importance on which one from their soul family will physically carry them to full term. It is just timing. When it comes to marriage and producing children, it is like a big conveyer belt. If the energies are right, whoever is there in that linear timeframe slips into that life slot. That is why you always draw in the same kind of partner type, different stories but still very similar. The Soul Window that opens during child bearing years make sure those partners become available. It dashes on the rocks the romantic and spiritual illusion of having the one ultimate soul mate in your life. My theory also does not make claim that a matriarchal child energetically mapped to the mother, does not have attachment to the father, they do. The parent not mapped to the child will experience love more on an environmental element than karmic coding. If they are there, loving and present, the child will bond. This is why you will have a child with a parent who has really bad parenting skills and the child still prefers that parent regardless of the treatment they receive. On the other hand, you will have a parent that would do anything for their child and they are almost ambivalent about that parent. This sometimes explains when divorce happens, you will see a parent able to walk away from nurturing their children while others fight tooth and nail to keep them in their lives at all cost. You can look at any family unit and see the matriarchal and patriarchal mapping with each child. It is all agreed upon before incarnation, so there are no bad guys or mistakes once the child has imprinted with a chosen parent.

So what are the scheduled life cycle signals for? Well the obvious is to guide and direct the soul to make changes as the soul's vehicle grows into maturity. These energetic life cycle signals open the Soul Windows. The dreaming soul awakens and makes the important choices on the next life cycle of your journey, then energetically re-maps and directs the beginning of something new. It is similar to having a new program downloaded into a computer. When the scheduled life cycle signal goes off and matches up with the present etheric life energies, it allows the soul to look through a Soul Window and see what changes are scheduled for the future. It is a plan of action that YOU wrote. It also allows the soul to make choices regarding those changes. That is what free will is about. At certain ages in our life, these life cycle signals go off and you are compelled to do something new, think something new, feel differently about yourself, your life or you now want different things. If we did not have these scheduled life cycle signals to direct us, regardless of being physically grown up, we would still be in an immature state of mind and emotions stuck in a perpetual life rerun. I sometimes made that point with clients that without these life cycle signals, you would be seeing grandmothers still carrying around their Barbie dolls as role models if not pushed for mature change. When that scheduled life cycle signal goes off, we outgrow the desires of one life cycle and want something different to be, to do, to have or to accomplish. The Soul Windows are part of that handbook we came into this life with to help

guide us on the journey we wrote but now do
not remember how it is suppose to turn out.

First Soul Window / The Awakening!

The first scheduled life cycle signal goes off around 6 years of age, which is actually the seventh year and will last until around 14 years of age. It is a minor Soul Window but where you begin to see a child start forming a definitive personality, wanting to do things their own way, express themselves differently and have definite opinions of what they like and do not like. It is where the child comes into the age of reasoning, making the first decisions based on what was written for their soul journey. You know the stances the young ones take:" I can do it myself, don't touch me, and leave me alone". They start becoming very independent thinkers. This scheduled life cycle signal begins to take form as a new soul identity. The soul discovers it now once again has a life that belongs only to them. This is when the soul is first aware they have choices in a new life to live and experience. The soul in the first few years of life has awareness and even some memory but does not have the maturity or power to make any changes in their external life. They are now capable of making their first choices how they will deal with the emotional responses to the environment around them. This is an approximate time line but some children will begin to exhibit these traits earlier. This happens from character coding, meaning an advantage in intelligence and birth sign influence.

The important thing always to remember is the soul chose their birth situation. Whatever emotions you are exposed to from the ages of 4 to 7 years of age will determine the belief system you will carry for the rest of your life. Whatever feeling definitions given to you for love, value, worth, judgment, and conditional behavior will shape all of your adult choices and sets the stage for addressing the soul's issues. At this age, your parents are the closest thing to a God definition you will ever identify within its purest form. You will love them unconditionally. You carry these feeling definitions without question at the beginning of this Soul Window. The child before this first Soul Window will just want to be loved and have their needs met. Most of those energetic traits will have dissipated when a child moves into the so-called terrible twos and threes. A child does not have the ability to discern how to make loving and moral choices before the age of seven, so if they see abusive behavior by you, that will be ok for them too because you do it. When the first Soul Window opens and before the opportunity to make life choices, the child will be like a sponge. The child will be whatever they are shown to be, told to be or in whatever manner they are treated, regardless of whether it is seemingly bad or good. If you teach a child, they are of no value or worthless, the child will naturally assume there is something lacking in them. If you abuse a child, they will think they did something to deserve it. The child feels every emotion, action and behavior in black or white terms. They are without the adult gray area of reason surrounding any action. In their innocence, they are incapable of blaming someone else for their misfortune. This life cycle creates the belief foundations for the Inner Child's guidance system of all your emotions and a subconscious program that will control responses for the rest of your life unless consciously changed. The first Soul Window will stay in place from approximately seven years to about 13 or 14 years of age. It is an age of emotional exploration and moves the child farther and farther away from maternal or paternal tethering. You can compare it to a puppy let out in the backyard for the first time...many, many adventures to be experienced in this new lifetime. The first few Soul Windows usually open very close together, getting farther apart as you get older with some rest periods in-between them.

HOW THE INNER CHILD CONTROLS YOU WITH "IT"

Before I move on to the second Soul Window, I would like to share some helpful information known in many areas of metaphysics and counseling as the Inner Child. Your divine self uses the Inner Child's emotional responses as a learning tool to help you grow and change. Through the years of counseling, I heard many clients famously use these phrases: "I know I should have done, said or stopped whatever <u>BUT</u> I love him, I need it, I can't do without him or it." "Even though I know I should, I just do not know why I don't or can't." These statements are all versions of the Inner Child's definition of an "IT". Another version of the "IT" is an unhealthy need for something outside of you: "If I only had that or when I get this, then I will be happy and feel good about myself or not feel ashamed, embarrassed and humiliated anymore". You can fill in the blanks on just about anything that you believe you need in order to be whole, feel safe, like and love yourself. Some people are clueless on what the concept would feel like not needing something to feel happy and content with who you are. Because of that, I often hear frustrated comments from successful women with everything going for them and still acting like begging little girls when it comes to men and relationships. The "IT" also creates a tendency to never being satisfied with anything gotten or accomplished by YOU. Your definition of self is less than, so nothing that YOU create in your life will compensate for that feeling. The key to recognizing those feelings is the banner cry of the Inner Child and summed up in this one word...BUT! A very powerful and manipulative dialogue used by the Inner Child to make you feel like crap! Everything before the word BUT is the adult trying to make sense of a ridiculous need and the frustrating choices you are forced into to get that need met. Everything after the word BUT is the Inner Child telling you exactly what it needs to feel safe, loved and happy and will make you compromise everything you are to give it to her. Just make a point of listening to your dialogue when you use the infamous word BUT and you will start recognizing the communications of your Inner Child's needs. The Inner Child's emotions are how the divine self communicates with you and the energetic child self never grows up. You do not actually want the Inner Child to grow up, as it is the foundation for the wonderment and joy in life experienced through a child's ability to believe anything is possible. In other words, hope and imagination used in manifesting your dreams! You also cannot allow the Inner Child's four-year-old emotions to control you for the rest of your life with bullying fear. The source of all this conflict begins with a full-blown temper tantrum your Inner Child lays on you. If you have ever seen a four year old having a temper tantrum, you know you can neither reason, threaten nor control their outpouring of distress. You must comply with her wishes or have earned a relationship of trust that you can guide her out of it. Unless you have that trust, inevitably you will have to give in to her because she will not give up until she gets her needs met. The experience of life to the Inner Child is comparable to walking through a dark forest in the scary unknown, knowing there are fearful things that will jump out and possibly hurt you. The Inner Child relies on you as the adult to overcome their fears with your soothing trust and values they can count on. She must be able to trust you to walk her through this journey knowing both of you will be ok. The adult can only do this if they have the knowledge of where the Inner Child's fear is coming from. You have to be able to get the Inner Child's acceptance that fear is only an illusion, something that goes bump in the night and she is safe with you. The challenge being the Inner Child's emotions and beliefs are so strong and powerful when filled with fear, they can overcome adult reasoning when faced with life's challenges. Those emotions are truly like a four year old, living only in a black and white world. She will either feel safe or afraid, feel loved or unloved, will trust or will trust nothing. The Inner Child does not have the ability like an adult to reason out in the gray area that we con ourselves into thinking we are in control or can manipulate situations and people.

The Inner Child only believes in the "IT", which will give her what she needs… love, safety, trust and happiness. The adult will then take the idea of the "IT" and turn it into mature themes of desperately needing to be married, being wealthy, being thin or being obsessively fixated on their career. Just pick something, anything and that will become the fixer. Of course, when you get that something, you will certainly find another something that will take "IT's" place. Similar to having in your closet at all times, all the latest pairs of fashionable shoes that shows everyone "you are so special"! Since the Inner Child is never satisfied with YOU or what YOU do give her, it is an on-going unfulfilling mission to get that

"IT" from outside of yourself to feel happy and satisfied.

I liked giving clients an affirmation called "Fake It Till You Make It" that seemed to appease the Inner Child and could actually calm the obsessive "IT" until it was addressed. The affirmation seemed to have the ability to give the Inner Child hope for a new and better future, which is how we learn to trust, heal and grow. This affirmation takes away the Inner Child's ability to allow her fears to paint you into a corner with no possible solutions. "IT" is the do or die feeling you get if you do not give her what she believes will make her happy. The affirmation is very effective and seems to calm the fears of abandonment and hopelessness. This is how it recites: "Regardless of what or how my situation may appear at the moment (fill in the blanks on your issue or challenge), regardless of how I feel about it at the moment (fill in the blanks with the appropriate emotions), I know without a doubt in my heart that everything will work out beautifully for me." "Why do I know this, because God has my back!"

I also gave an additional ending when there were issues about needing a particular person in their life in order to be happy. It went something like this: "Thank you God and all the divine powers that be for this wonderful experience of having this man or woman in my life." "I am in complete gratitude for having the opportunity to share with this person regardless of the experience, as I know that I have learned and grown from it." "If he or she is the right person for me then somehow or someway, I will be shown this clearly." "If this person is not right for my happiness, I know without a doubt the wonderful relationship with a beautiful, caring and loving partner will be coming into my life right behind." "Thank you." Very effective and soothing for the Inner Child believing there is someone to hope for if this relationship does not work out. Hope is the key word here. As long as the Inner Child has hope for an unknown future, she will begin to let go of the obsessive "IT" that paints you into a corner to get what she or he thinks will make both of you happy right now.

I personally have always asked the divine powers to make my messages very clear. I happen to like seeing an energetic billboard somewhere in my mind, as I can be a little dense. I am one of those learners who do not do subtle or vague well when trying to shift perception. It is one of those little quirks you are designed with, having your finest quality also your so-called Achilles heel. I am extremely persistent in getting the answers I want when making changes but that same wonderful quality also makes me stubborn and resistant to change. Not knowing when it is time to let go and let God. Go Figure! I found a lot of resistance in clients when I gave that affirmation to those addicted to feeling the pain of disappointment and then the wonderful relief when it goes away. It can be very seductive. When you have finally gotten over a heartbreak or disappointment, it is a powerful, manipulative and illusory tool used by the ego to create the same scenario over and over again just so you can experience that wonderful temporary relief it brings. It would be in the same category as doing drugs, drinking binges, smoking, excessive shopping sprees or sex addiction. It makes you feel powerful and temporarily good about yourself when you can make those addictions go away for a time. Inevitably, you want to feel it again. If you are not powerful from within, regardless of the external discipline, you will repeat the addictive behavior in order to feel that relief. You win this tug of war with your Inner Child by re-confirming to yourself over and over again, that a miracle and a solution will come through that doorway at any moment! Believe! Believe! Believe! This affirmation is a big help with people who worry a lot about trying to control future outcomes. The only control you really have in your life are what emotions you are going to choose to deal with any situation. Those emotions in the now moment is creating your future. Once you realize this, you become very observant and very careful about what you think and feel about any situation.

SECOND SOUL WINDOW / THIS LIFE IS MINE!

The second Soul Window opens around 14 or 15 years of age and continues through around the ages of 21 or so. It is hard to determine exact age as timelines are designed by agreement of the soul and the divine self, like a fingerprint of identity. Each one is unique for that soul. Also what makes it hard to pin down the exact timing of spiritual energetics, as our age is always a year ahead of what we call a birthday. When we say we are 14 years of age, we are actually in our 15th year of life. So bear with me on the approximate age of the Soul Windows. This second Soul Window is one of the most tumultuous and challenging next to the one called Chiron Return (50th return year), which is generally labeled mid-life crisis. At this point, the soul is in the energetics similar to a new colt trying out its running legs. This Soul Window brings the big bang of self-awareness! This is when the 14 or 15 year old goes into the hormonal insanity of being a teenager. They have all the doubts, new feelings and new awareness that their life should belong only to them. You have a volcanic energetic awakening that looks like "My life, my body, my way!" If you have not given strong foundations of rolling with the flow to your offspring, you have one strung out temperamental soul having a power surge of new life discovery! They have to walk the energetic balance beam of being in awe of their new journey but they must also be taught respect; honoring themselves and others. The drive of wanting to do their life exactly the way they want to do it is sometimes overwhelming and of course, that is when parental guidance comes big into play. The soul's energy is in hyper-overdrive believing they can leap off high buildings, drive 100 miles an hour, drink a fifth of whiskey and do drugs without any consequence of paying the price or getting caught. You can compare this energetic shift to the scene in the movie of Home Alone, when the young child discovers he has the whole house to himself and can do anything he wants! They are hypersensitive and plugged in full tilt to all new emotions and feelings of false power. It feels fabulous and horrible at the same time. They are over the top and cannot get enough! This is the Soul Window where future consequences are rarely taken into account. One of them being the young adult believes they will never get old like their parents! This particular Soul Window stays open until around 19 years to 21 years. It does eventually calm down, thank God! It is an extremely tough time for parenting to learn how to walk between setting the boundaries of authority and being compassionate to their child's journey. This is the time you will see mirrored back to you as a parent in bright neon lights the old saying, "The fruit never falls too far from the tree". Your children will be wonderful gifts to you, mirroring back your own issues you also came to address in life.

Energetic Neutral Zones

Once you start reaching maturity, you begin to experience what I call neutral zones or time outs. This is where you give yourself the time to process new energetic mappings, rest for awhile and get ready for the new round of change scheduled in the next Soul Window opening. It is similar to an energetic cork bobbing in the water, becoming balanced and preparing to put new programs into place. Sometimes these down times are the most challenging as you move into your mature years. Our egos are not the most patient, waiting for future results. You can make some pretty big changes emotionally, mentally, spiritually and in your life arena in these neutral zones. As usual, you want to make something happen on YOUR timetable. This neutral zone is sometimes viewed as a stalemate in your life where nothing seems to be moving fast enough for you. You are bored and feel as though what you want to happen will never come about. These neutral zones will happen many times in your life. It seems there is no set schedule between which Soul Windows this takes place for you, or how many times. You put these neutral zones into place to prepare for the next Soul Window and to process energetic changes already taking place. Some are created for a rest period to let the so-called dust settle after a particularly challenging growth, some are created to rev up energetic patterns to get ready to start something big and new and some are created as a deep contemplative time to go within and listen to your inner guidance. Regardless of why you created them, most of the time they seem to generate a frustrating and impatient feeling of being bored and unfulfilled in your life. Sometimes these neutral zones can be scarier than the changes before and after. They can bring an intense feeling of nothingness, which our humanity is not designed to deal well with for a reason. Change is to be constantly on the table for us. They can be particularly intense with young adults and then once again at mid-life. One should be very watchful not to allow the impatient Inner Child to paint you into an "IT" corner while in these frustrating waiting times. You designed them to catch your breath and make a new game plan. If you let your ego (Inner Child's emotional tantrums) willfully push you into forcing change before you are ready, it is usually a wasted effort. The neutral zones are a good place to learn and practice going with the flow and learning how to trust in the process. Patience is the big keyword here!

Third Soul Window / Making Grown Up Future Choices

The third Soul Window opens around 22 thru 30 years of age. This marks the beginning of identifying what your definitions of maturity will be. Usually, this is where you will see the first neutral zone between Soul Windows. It leaves a time-period of a few years where you do not know what you want to be when you grow up and/or really not interested in growing up all. You would like to have all the adult compensations without any of the responsibilities. Please remember, all ages are approximate and everyone's life storyline is different, like a fingerprint. This Soul Window is where the desire to make your first adult decisions are presented to you by choice or you have them forced upon you by the script you wrote. Your first realization you have the power to do what you want and your life journey really does belong to you. You now also begin to understand your life choices have long-term effects. You may have made some of the same choices when you were in the previous Soul Window of 15 to 21 years but now it becomes very apparent that you are feeling differently about them. You begin to feel the guilt, regret and victim energy about those young choices and can begin to blame others for the state of your life. In the previous awakening Soul Window, you just are not aware and perceptive to the effects of what you do in relationship to others. You truly are only concerned about your needs and really do not understand the long-term future consequences of those choices. This is where you start contemplating making those long-term future decisions by the seat of your pants. This Soul Window is where you can make the most seemingly bad choices from impulsive decisions. Unless of course you cookie cutter and prototype your life after your parents in the need for parental approval. Then you have a whole other life script that eventually has to be dealt with, as you must one day map your own journey, usually in midlife crisis. You are still in a Soul Window of hedonistic gratification and immediate nurturing to feel good. That is why most marriages that bond before 30 in these energetic tumultuous times do not make it unless both partners energetically and spiritually grow together. You make decisions based on that he is really handsome, I like the way he dresses, he has great friends, he drives an expensive car and he makes me laugh versus is he going to be a good father, good provider and how does he independently walk his own journey? In this Soul Window, you feel the "life itch". You begin to feel restless, bored, and unhappy with childish and immature things that once made you happy. You are ready to bring about change in your life based around the choices of long-term future commitments such as having children, changing careers, getting married and buying a home. These are your first conscious adult decisions building your future. I say adult decisions but that does not necessary mean wise or mature decisions. If you designed a journey to learn what being fearless is about, you will make many not so good choices and do-overs. You will experience repeatedly, the emotions of failure so you can get past the fear and judgment of it. In the big scheme of your soul's journey, it all means nothing! You are going to get there this lifetime or in the next 100 lifetimes but you will ultimately arrive, aware and enlightened!

FOURTH SOUL WINDOW / OMG! I JUST FOUND A WRINKLE!

This Soul Window opens up between the ages of 32 to around 38 years, give or take a year or two. This is what I call the "tumbling tower" Soul Window. It is where you reevaluate all your young adult choices. This is the age group where you see so many marriages fall apart after 7 to 10 years. You make the choice if something is not working, you decide to get rid of it, or make some serious life adaptations to compensate for the unhappiness. If something is not making you happy, you move on, find a substitute or decide if you are going to mask the pain and unhappiness with anything to deaden the hurt and frustration you feel about your life. Maturity creeps up on you whether you like it or not, even if wisdom does not follow. We start looking at the choices and decisions we made in our 20's, asking if those choices will hold in the future of your soul's journey. This Soul Window is where you re-evaluate everything in your life; nothing is spared....family, marriage, having children, career, health, aging, and friends. Whatever your soul's script has prioritized is what will come up the strongest and demand the most attention.

Some people in this Soul Window decide to take a pass on the first big free will opportunity and do whatever it takes to make it go away or substitute it with a new and improved version of the same problem. This is just different packaging, like bouncing from one same relationship or job with different players in your arena. In the previous energetic earth push before the Aquarius age we are in now, we could put this Soul Window off until our 50's or 60's. Then it came on with a vengeance, what everyone calls a mid-life crisis. In the present earth energetics, this is not possible. Everything is moving very quickly now, almost instantaneously. We are seeing issues demanding to be resolved much sooner than in the past. If you take a pass, you will not see it disappear and settle into the dust until you get older as the old patterns allowed. You will see the issue come up again almost immediately, sometimes relentlessly until action is taken. That is why so many people are feeling overwhelmed with old issues they thought were gone and buried or never wanted to deal with them in the first place. Those issues will not go away and now you are not able to stick your head in the sand to escape them. You have to take the responsibility for the life journey you wrote or your written script will do it for you.

A good indicator you are being pushed into change is when you can make a statement something of the sort; "Wow, didn't see that coming!" This is how the divine self gets your attention! It begins with a little emotional nudge of thoughts and feelings that you know you should change and correct something important in your life. If you do not ask the hard questions of...WHAT?, then it starts feeling like a little marble rolling around in your mind and just keeps popping up again and again. Sometimes what needs to be addressed is rather obvious and then sometimes not so obvious. Thoughts keep coming up like: "I really need to do this, start this, leave this, change this." It just will not go away! These are the signals that it is time to start cleaning out the proverbial closet of imbalanced karma or heavy emotional baggage that keeps you from experiencing life to the fullest and being in joy.

If you still do not do anything about those subtle messages, your divine self will step up the nudging to energetic and emotional shoving situations, causing you to feel it is getting pretty obvious and so in your face that change is needed. For example, you have had a nice or maybe not so nice job that you have been meaning to leave for a few years and try something new or go back to school but just have not made the move for this or that reason. What happens at this point is all of a sudden, you get a new boss from hell! Now the energy is like a tack on your seat and becomes an uncomfortable situation, aggravating you on a steady basis. It is now something you cannot ignore and shove into a closet by creating diversions; instead you are being properly shoved by your divine self. Finally if you do not pay attention to the nudging and the consistent shoving experiences of having it right in your face, your divine self basically takes the energetic attitude of "OK, you won't make a choice, let the changes begin!" Your divine self boots you out! That is where you get the proverbial rug pulled out from under you. It is not one of those circumstances where you can say, "Wow, I did not see that coming"! All the signs have been there talking to you. You just made the choice to ignore them. When that situation has drastically changed, you are now forced to make choices one way or the other. You are fired, laid off from the job you have hated or have been bored with for years. Your partner chooses someone else in their life after years of an unhappy situation between the two of you. A health matter comes to surface in a much more serious tone than it would have before because you ignored the symptoms. You must now make those changes in your life, regardless of past decisions. It is at this point the only option in front of you is how you are going to address them. You can be in victim mode or ask for the divine assistance of strength to get through the challenge. You keep hope of a powerful and positive outcome through your faith and prayer. There is a big difference in the outcome of any situation based on what your choice will be.

Still nothing is being done TO you, your divine self is part of who you are and you have agreed to this on some level. IT IS ALL YOU! These changes are going to happen one way or another since you wrote them before entering into this life adventure. You might as well do them on your own conscious terms instead of being not so gently reminded that you did make the agreement. This is always the choice of free will. You will design the journey, the players and the tools that show up. How you choose to experience the journey is always up to you, whether you make the decision to change freely or be pushed into it. One way or the other change will come. It is you, who decides if the changes come in power or weakness. You are the one who designed this game and you are the one who makes the choice for change. No one can do that for you, even as hard as you try to pass it off on others. You always have choices in this virtual reality game called life: to make this a Disneyland experience or a nightmare....it is your call. Just remember when you are designing your life from wherever it is we rest between these incarnations: experiencing a hurricane, auto wreck, loss of a loved one, health crisis or any other seemingly hard luck challenge seemed like a pretty good idea when writing your soul's learning script. You decide it is just the tool needed to accomplish your life journey. Your divine self is completely detached to what your choices are, just making sure the choices come about as you agreed and wrote them for this lifetime. The challenges WILL come but the important factor for growth is, how are you going to deal with them? Are you going to go directly to negative victim mode of blame, anger and helplessness or are you going to persevere with faith and the inner strength of knowing that you can weather anything with the help of that divine part of you. If you take the higher road, regardless of how things may appear at any given moment and have faith they will get better, then you WILL be ok. Even if at that moment, you cannot see a way out. I will say that most of the dramatic changes that come about in this Soul Window are usually a much milder version of what energetically happens in the Sixth Soul Window, which is the most powerful Soul Window you created...Mid Life Crisis! It is always better to get a jump-start on major life changes in this Soul Window in preparation for the next two. The next Soul Window giving you the first good look at your mortality, yikes! The following Soul Window of Chiron Return is the window that is relentless in intensity and the biggest and most powerfully reactive of all windows.

LIVING IN MULTIPLE DIMENSIONS

The discovery of Soul Windows brought about another obvious fact for me that we are constantly in dimensional flux. We change and grow in gradual shifts of perceptions and time lines. We are emotionally reacting from past events, experiencing life in the present and creating future experiences all at the same time. This was the most difficult concept for me to grasp, living your life on multiple dimensions at the same time. I think this is important to bring up before we move on to the next Soul Window as this window shows many of the effects of this peculiarity. This multidimensional life concept has been written about by many spiritual teachers, although personally I thought they might be dipping into too much happy weed when I first read about it. It just drove me a little crazy because I could not get my mind around it and I consider myself relatively intelligent. I finally understood the concept or think I have to an extent I can explain it in layman's terms without all the ethereal metaphysical woo-woo definitions. It was after reading a few new books and pondering on the new Soul Window information that it started to make some sense.

When we go through challenges in life, it is for one reason and one reason only, we are here to release the emotional baggage we have been carrying that keeps us from being completely connected to Oneness. There are always different versions of ourselves that we are experiencing at the same time. The self that is still in negative fear and trying to work through an issue, the self that sees glimpses of being free of the fear with the desire to grow and the self that is completely fearless the majority of the time. As you awaken and let go of old issues, you can simultaneously live in several dimensions and experience various versions of you at the same time. That is why you sometimes seem to have gotten over an issue but then you find yourself sliding back to being the old way and then finally breaking through. When you do this, you are another version of you living a completely different life because that version of you no longer has that issue. We even use the phrases, "when I used to be like that or that was the old me". Well, where did the old you go? That old you is existing in a life dimension where your negative fear is and the new you is living in a reality without it. It is still all you just several different versions of you simultaneously existing at the same time. You will also hear people make the innocent statement when pointing out they do not live like that or experience something they do not relate to, "Not in my world, that does not happen"! What they are really saying is even though they exist in your world with you at that moment, your drama does not exist for them in their world or dimension. You are sharing a space in time but not the same energetic dimensional beliefs. It is very tricky but important to understand how powerful your ability is to create your world and environment by your thoughts and beliefs, both past, present and future.

With every choice you make for change, you literally re-design your life to become something else that also changes the world you exist in. While in the process of those changes, you can literally have one foot in the dimension of the old way and one foot in the world of your new creation. If you stay positive in every choice coming before you, it can make all the difference in an extremely challenging situation. You must accept that whatever energy you put into a situation or a life choice will recreate and reflect back to you in some form. If you go all victim, negative, bitching, complaining, blaming, crying the blues over your misfortune, you will only see more people in your life that relate to those situations. If you can take a challenging situation, regardless of how it has the potential for spiraling down into fear and stay steadily focused on a safe outcome for you, things will always change for the better. By that, I mean being in complete faith, trust and accepting that everything will turn out all right. For example, when the four destructive hurricanes came through Florida, my home was directly in the path of all four. We were literally untouched, though surrounded by a circle of damage through my neighborhood. Four times the winds and rain somehow always seemed to be a little less terrible where my home was. I of course had family in other states praying for my safety. Why I believe we went through those hurricanes without incident was the attitude of everyone who was in my home at the time. We absolutely kept the conversation on how there was going to be minimal or no damage to our home and we were going to be perfectly safe. All day we also kept sending good thoughts to everyone else. We were only out of electricity for a half a day and never went without water. Our positive beliefs created a safe dimension where the hurricane would not cause extensive damage to our home. Because of those powerful beliefs, the chaos swirled around us. The surrounding homes all had extensive storm damage. Those homes matched their fear and belief of the hurricane's destructive force.

So make your choice, creating a sad, gloomy future of more worry, lack and fear or one of a brighter future with hope, optimism and faith. As we did with the hurricanes, embracing the absolute knowing that somehow everything was going to be ok. I can guarantee you not one moment did I think I could control those roaring winds or torrential rains. What I did know was that I was completely not interested in getting slammed by them. The people around me that experienced extensive damage to their homes were focused on the fear of just that. What you put your energy into; you draw into your dimensional existence. My neighbors experienced those hurricanes through what their beliefs told them was possible and I experienced what my beliefs told me. Personally, I was happy with the reality I created of not having to re-shingle my roof or sweep up plate glass out of my home.

FIFTH SOUL WINDOW / FEELING OUR MORTALITY

This particular Soul Window is what I call the Preparation Window, experienced from the ages of 39 to around 45 years of age. It also includes some of the most intense neutral zones during your soul's journey. These years help make preparation and give you a heads up on Chiron Return, which is the biggest and most powerful Soul Window on your journey. During this particular Soul Window and the approximate years within, you begin to feel the tug of aging and for the first time become aware of your own mortality. Regardless of anyone's obsession with holding the aging process off with super creams or all the available cosmetic surgery of nip and tuck, we become acutely aware that we are going to get old. The idea that one day you will leave this life does not really enter into the equation of what you are trying to accomplish until you hit this Soul Window. You begin to experience the little pull towards feeling older and facing in real time that you are no longer considered part of the youth culture. If you have based your whole existence on everything outside yourself: career, looks, money or social standing, this is where the realization begins that you are now competing with younger people for your job, dates or attention. For the first time you feel invisible because of your age group. What you used to get with your fresh good looks and vivaciousness you now have to barter with power or control. The younger generation begins to take the spotlight away from you and most of us get really offended by this process. Hollywood is a perfect example of this kind of animal. When you are talented, fresh, young and under 35 years of age, you have a decent chance of catching the eye of some kind of production. If you have not made your mark by then, you can very quickly go from an A lister or never even making it to the alphabet. In this Soul Window, the first moment you become mam or sir, you are usually taken aback by it. Mostly, you do not like it!

I remember the first time being called mam; I was so stunned that I thought the young guy was talking to someone else. I mean after all, I still looked good at that age and when I realized he WAS talking to me, I pretty much felt like I wanted to slap the kid for just a second or two. Thank God, I am a pacifist these days, leaving my wild temper back in my 20's and 30's. I still chuckle about my daughter hitting her 40's and every time she would talk to me about things like menopause, make up for the mature skin and so on, her voice always took on the hushed whisper of disbelief as though there was a mistake going on. You KNOW that whisper, the kind people use when they are addressing an uncomfortable topic with you. I mean after all, she was a hip San Francisco woman, tattooed, very cool mom and wife with a successful career. It couldn't be happening to her! I know she had the big aversion in having to get her mind and emotions wrapped around the idea of now being looked at as a mature woman, as we all do. You know, like her mom for God's sake! I tried to reassure her that going into the aging years and exhibiting menopausal symptoms was not a bad word that she had to whisper about, it happened to every woman regardless. Personally, I do not think she bought it, as I also remember not wanting to buy the aging crap either.

This Soul Window resembles a pre-sale, giving you the opportunity to make preparations getting the best bargain for your next life challenge. You also will lay down more of the necessary and helpful groundwork that will make the next Soul Window of Chiron Return easier. You start getting rumblings that you did not get exactly what you wanted out of life or did get and accomplish everything you thought you wanted but have now discovered an emptiness feeling something like "Is that all there is"? Other rumblings feel like this: you always wanted a successful career and have accomplished it but never even gave a thought to having or even wanting children. Now you find you cannot take your eyes off newborn babies and kids. Oh my God, now you realize you really want children and that fabulous career is wonderful but not everything! Other changes will be career dissatisfaction, leaving long time partners and choosing other lifestyles. Anything that you begin to realize you are dissatisfied with or feel you are lacking in life. It comes up as doubt, questioning and asking yourself some hard questions about your life choices such as: what if, what if and what if? No one escapes it, but what you decide to do with this opportunity is of course free will. You can take this pre-sale offer or take a pass and then wait for the inevitable full on shake your life up awakening of the dreaming soul in the next Soul Window.

I would like to add that gender is not a factor when this happens. Gender only brings about different emotional choices and tools you come in with to use. The male gender is not designed to mature as fast or the same as women. It is always an energetic female issue, meaning men have underlying imprints of being a hunter and breadwinner so nurturing oneself does not come naturally as with women. When a soul decides to come into a life incarnation as a man or a woman with strong male tendencies, it is because learning how to nurture and have compassion is usually the main agenda. Female gender comes by nurturing naturally, as it is a feminine energy. Of course, there are always exceptions since there are really no set rules to follow during this Disney adventure. The foundations of the soul's journey unfold exactly the same way for both genders. We make those choices of learning to nurture ourselves by playing the roles of the tough little boy or the adorable little girl and everything else in between. You are here to experience your chosen path, to grow emotionally and spiritually. We grow, we change and then we awaken to the inevitable truth that we are God beings and of Oneness.

So basically the late 30's and early 40's are the years of "what if?", would have, should have or the could have questions on choices you have already made or have not yet made. You find yourself making statements to yourself and others that you are not getting old, you are cool, and you can still party with the best of them. Then one day you realize, astounded and a little horrified when you hear yourself making a comment about "those 20 or 30 year olds" doing this or that. You have just been completely blindsided by your youth slipping away. Of course, we hang on to those hip, young thinking outlooks for a little longer until one day you make the startling discovery that you do not feel comfortable with your skirt 6 inches above your knees or your Doc Martin boots do not go with your suits. Aaaaah, the glories of youth now gone! OMG! This window pretty much centers completely around the realization that you are NOT going to be 25 for the rest of your life, so now what do you do with that?

Every soul's journey is of course different with many aspects coming into play such as astrological birth sign influence, genetics and the ease or difficulty of the challenge you wrote for yourself. These influences have a great deal of impact on whether you will be aggressive or take a wait see attitude on the coming Chiron Return Soul Window. You may choose to make the decision to get a jumpstart and bring into motion many of the inevitable changes and challenges presented in the next Soul Window. There is always a feeling of uncertainty as to why you are making these changes in your life; you just know they need to be done. You may also hold your breath awhile for the soul to fully awaken and start changing your life with or without any preparation. It is like taking a test you are hoping to pass, if you study and prepare it will be easier. If you do not, you address the changes sliding in by the seat of your pants and hope you get it right. Regardless of what or how you choose, change will happen both internally and in your life environment. There is no right way or wrong way to address this Soul Window in preparation, there is only your way. After this Soul Window, you go into one of those down times, a resting mode to ponder decisions made or not made. You take the deep breath before the big leap that represents getting to the top of the mountain and the beginning of the coasting, adjusting and reclaiming portion of your life.

SIXTH SOUL WINDOW / CHIRON RETURN...A RESET AND DO-OVER!

This is the most powerful and largest Soul Window, when the dreaming soul fully awakens and evaluates your life situation. It usually starts around 46 or 47 and will sometimes continue at late as 67 years of age, depending on how large your life agenda is. Now is when you get energetically re-mapped to finish or possibly begin to accomplish what you came here to experience. You get a chance to reset or create a do-over in every area of your life, if you choose to do so. Some people's Chiron Return (the 50-year birth cycle) is a big time-frame lasting onward to 15 years or so but most are around 8 or 9 years if some of the release work was done in the previous Soul Windows. It also depends on how big the life challenge is you are unfolding. This is the window notoriously famous for "poking the sleeping bear" energy. If you had not addressed the long deeply buried issues coming to the surface before in another Soul Window, it is particularly intense and usually pulls the rug right out from under your feet in some area of your life. The dreaming soul looks around and asks the question of self: "Am I happy, am I fulfilled with who and what I perceive myself to be, do I feel joy, have I done what I came here to do?" If you have done the preliminary work in the previous Soul Window in your 40's and addressed some of your life issues, this window can be a completion of those awakenings. If not, then the issues pretty much come flying at you with an intensity that can make you feel you are losing your sanity. Unfortunately, in dealing with these intense emotions, our medical society loves to issue little pills to make it all go away. We are supposed to feel those emotions, it is a sign that our divine self is pushing for change. Some of the hard issues that may come up are quitting a successful career to follow a lifelong dream or realizing you do not want to be married to the person you have spent half your life with. All of a sudden big health issues show up and of course, the powerful spiritual questions will come up about life and why are we actually here? You may do some really stupid things like getting involved in an affair with a 22 year old or make some wonderful monumental decisions like finally deciding to go back to school and get your degree. You may not know why you are thinking and feeling the emotions and thoughts but they are there with an intensity you cannot ignore. These changes are only tools to help you see what underlying issues need to be addressed. Whatever it is, it is unfinished business of the soul. Depending on personality type, you may suddenly do some quick stopping and brand new starts or it may take years of slowly cooking like a crock-pot. There is no set rule for anyone, only the imprinted journey you designed for yourself. It is only YOU who has designed this journey and responsible for making those choices.

Chiron Return is a long Soul Window as you are making decisions about how to wrap things up in this incarnation. I have rarely counseled anyone with a short Soul Window addressing Chiron Return. This Soul Window is where some foundation of spirituality comes in handy, a lot would be better. When the foundations of your virtual reality game called life begin to come into question, this is where you make the choice if you are seriously going to go within or only make superficial changes on the outside. If you have not listened to your divine inner voice prompting you, not been kind to yourself, not made yourself a priority in your own life journey, not loved yourself enough, not addressed your spiritual self or whatever it is that you should have done or not have done....all holy hell breaks loose!! Change begins to happen whether you are ready for it or not! The energy on earth right now is extremely high intensity, pushing the ascension journey of all souls with almost instantaneous results from your sub-conscious belief systems. Everything is coming fast and hard, manifesting in such a way so you cannot miss it. In the past, you had the luxury of spending a few or many lifetimes working on an important issue you needed to be free of. Not so anymore, you do not have 10 or 15 years to decide whether you are ready to make crucial life changes. You are either going to get it or you are going to reincarnation summer school to catch up. Everyone is destined to return home and no soul is left behind in the fabricated hell we have been taught to believe exists. The souls who are embracing the new consciousness will do everything to bring along all the souls who are still in old paradigms. I have noticed in counseling that many marriage contracts are now ending, one partner being more spiritually enlightened and married to a partner who is dragging a lot of ego. One partner given the opportunity to help raise a partnering soul by the exposure to their lighter energy and they either got or did not. Many less enlightened partners are being left behind at their level, the more enlightened partner needing to be free as the karmic contract is done. Imagine it this way, the more enlightened soul must fold in their energy like an angel would fold in their wings to exist in heavier human energies and then once the contract is fulfilled, the wings unfold and they begin to live life on their own terms. Now by no means, am I saying we are dealing with angels partnered with us to help our souls ascend, it was just a metaphor. I happen to like them, a lot!

It is also important to understand about this Soul Window that it aggravates the ego into full on hysteria. The ego does not like change at all, any kind of change where you take away the routine anchoring from your life. Your ego would rather have you stay in an unhappy familiar life situation where you know how to deal with the pain, recovery, pain, recovery routine than move onto something you cannot control... the future. But we are here to change, grow and experience God through YOU as YOU, in whatever scenario you have decided to create your life around. Think of it in the simple terms of experiencing God through your own experiences. Whatever they may be, they are still God experiencing through YOU. The big picture evolution will be your choices during that experience. Are you going to play the victim and walk on a path of self-judgment, blame, anger, bitterness, resentment, shame and humiliation? The other choice would be to allow the emotions and feelings of trust and faith in the divine outcome of all things, demonstrating compassion and kindness for you. Even when you screw up, you can be in gratitude for the smallest gift that comes out of the situation. The one thing most people miss in their spiritual evolution is the art of gratitude. Even the smallest gift is something that should be acknowledged and make it overshadow any negative circumstances in the moment. It is a difficult discipline and a skill that only comes with repeated practice. Remember your divine self is experiencing everything through you but your free will is in charge. That small voice you hear is your spiritual rah, rah divine cheerleader, urging you on to make an emotional choice to feel good about yourself. I gave clients a rule of thumb to recognize who is making your emotional decisions, your fear based ego stuck in the "but what ifs" or your divine self that whispers continuously that everything will be alright if you just have faith and believe. That rule of thumb is, if your thoughts and emotions do not make you feel good and makes you fearful, your ego is making choices from that place. If you feel good about doing the right thing, no matter how hard it may be, your divine self is trying to get you to step into your authentic Muchness to take responsibility and control of your life.

It is that information I always liked to share with clients to help them understand when their divine self has taken over this particular phase of the Soul Window. If you have an event in your life that you can make this statement: "Wow, I never saw that coming!", and you feel blindsided by the event whether it be challenging or joyous, then you know your ego has been pushed aside, bound and gagged of all whining and protest and your divine self is now in the drivers seat. You must not look at challenging events as punishment or that you have made some kind of life mistake. Even the most spiritually awakened souls are having a few severe crises going on in their life in this accelerated energy now on earth. It is a cleansing process and unfortunately, there is no lamb's blood "home free" symbol that gets marked on the door to pass you by as all other less enlightened folks out there go through hell. If it comes up as disease, disappointment, rage, sudden deaths, your life crumbling around you, then your divine self deems it necessary for you to experience those challenges to get the lesson. Remembering that your divine self is following a script you wrote. Of course, it is always free will in what choice you are going to make dealing with being unexpectedly blindsided. These are often life situations where you are left with no other choice but to deal with the reality before you. A husband leaving a wife of 25 years in a seemingly happy marriage, a successful business person selling everything and retiring to the beach to paint at the age of 54, leaving behind everyone and everything that were the trappings of his success. Good health throughout your life and now diagnosed with cancer or just cannot put your finger on what is wrong but you are no longer happy with your life and you feel sort of DEAD!

As you are experiencing these challenges, you must always remember there is no right way or wrong way. The only choice you have at that moment is how YOU are going to deal with it emotionally: positive or negative. This is free will and the real power you have over your life. There is no ONE or no THING that can take your right or ability to choose how you think, feel or believe about any circumstances created in your life arena. Based on the premise that YOU are creating every moment of it, then you must accept that what you are now experiencing is the results of your thoughts, beliefs and feelings created at some distant past and has now caught up with you. Your choices being: are you going to continue creating the life lessons needed to get the message you came here to learn in continuous negative drama or make it at the very least an enjoyable and exciting adventure. The reality is you are going to keep on trying until you finally understand that you are not separate from the divine or any other being you are sharing this experience with. No one can do your life for you and everyone else you are interacting with in your play can only view the event from their dimensional perspective. No one can do your dis-ease or death for you, no matter how famous, how wealthy or how loved you are. You cannot pay, beg, plead, force or accept an offer of exchange to take it from you. It is under those life circumstances that can really bring the intense fear up to the surface when you realize those facts and sometimes that miracle of faith.

So, you end up finishing this Soul Window, either with a total life refit, addressing what you could or maybe still dragging with you what you could not. At the very least, stuck your head in the sand and hoped that it would go away. Whatever choice you have made will come along with you into the next Soul Windows. Your life is now beginning to wind down and you are on the downside of the proverbial life mountain. The Soul Windows from this point get shorter, more profound and more deeply life altering. These changes will happen from the inside and outside, in preparation for your final life exam.

REMAINING SOUL WINDOWS / UNTIL WE GO HOME

After you have experienced the Chiron Return Soul Window, you immediately experience one of those neutral zones. It is always the roughest and most profoundly challenging of all of our Soul Windows and the energetic rest is definitely needed. The remaining Soul Windows will start shortly after Chiron Return window ends from around 62 or 63 years of age until passing. You will see the rest of your life unfold based on what choices you made going into these last Soul Windows. If you have unloaded many life contracts and swept away a lot of karmic bull crap, you will have a profound sense of freedom you may have never felt before. You have an intense feeling of not wanting responsibility for anyone but yourself. Getting close to retirement, you may make different choices on what that will look like: selling big homes and looking to travel light. You get on a new health program, wanting to stay more active. The heavy-duty emotional life choices you made in the previous Soul Window will program how you will spend the last chapters of your life…being vital and alive or sipping cold Campbell soup in a smelly nursing home, feeling useless, bitter and filled with regret. As the years slip by, depending on what death window you will choose (oh yes, we also design several death windows as an escape hatch if we decide we put too much on our plate in this life) the Soul Windows come in smaller, closer together and with less intensity. They are designed to be gentler but still urging and pushing to make at least some of the changes and learning lessons you came here to accomplish. Your divine self takes the approach if you missed the big boat in the last several Soul Windows, we are going to make it a little easier for you. We are still going to send a boat for you but now it is a smaller rowboat and if you still do not want to do any of the work, your divine self will send someone to row it for you. This comes from the saying it is never too late, even on deathbed release. The Soul Windows never stop opening until you take your last breath to give you the opportunity to make a choice of releasing old baggage and embracing unconditional love for self and others. The whole purpose of this adventure you call your life is to not bring with you to the next incarnation any of the karmic baggage you came into this life to unload.

How Our Beliefs Define Soul Windows

The one consistent rule addressing all the Soul Windows is you must listen to that small, insistent inner voice that speaks to you. You do this in quietness, whether it is in meditation or just nature walks. It is what calms the chatter of the conscious mind where the ego rules. The other indications that your divine self is trying to communicate with you is the fearful pit in the stomach, butterflies in the solar plexus, anxiety attacks, embarrassment, quick and unexpected anger or hurt. Your emotions are tools of divine self that communicates change is needed, giving you the opportunity to ask why you are feeling a certain way. Once again, the rule of thumb is if you think a thought, say something or are getting ready to make a choice, and it does not make you feel grounded, safe and happy, then don't do it or say it. Your ego is manipulating the Inner Child, trying to control something outside of yourself. The emotions you are experiencing in that moment are based on a belief you can actually control the experience you are having from outside of you. You are getting ready to compromise an authentic choice of self-love in order to feel those needed emotions at any cost and I do mean at ANY cost.

If you make a decision, say something or do something that gives you a good feeling about yourself, then your divine self is patting you on the back. It may not be an easy decision for you, it may even be a controversial decision but ultimately if you feel good about what has transpired, then you are on the right track. The ego will try to trick you into thinking that feeling self-righteous is the same thing. This is where working on your Muchness and having a personal "Tude" comes in handy. Knowing you have the right to think what you want and do what you want because you are willing to take full responsibility for those thoughts and actions. I am not talking about false pride or arrogance based on the need to be right, it is when you just know you have done the right thing for yourself and having compassion for all the participating characters. This is where most people have the hardest time distinguishing between the Inner Child's demand of "It's All About Me" and the divine self's "What About Me". I will explain the difference between these two emotions because they are deceptively very much alike.

When the Inner Child is in the energy of, "It's All About Me, It's All About Me, there is no YOU and I mean that seriously! Every action, every word, every nicety, every sacrifice, every moment of giving, loving, nurturing or buying is about manipulating the players in your life play to get the Inner Child's needs met from outside of you. Your life fills up with compromise, giving to get, resentment, jealousy, bitching and complaining about how no one seems to make you a priority in life. Whether done in suffering silence and you whine and complain only in your mind or you are blasting everyone, the results are the same. The passive version of this is the ultimate victim, being a wuss, whiny, manipulative, fawning, excessively shy, fearful and with anger always just bubbling under the surface. These soft, passive creatures have claws and they usually cover them up with major niceness. The aggressive version is much easier to spot, as they are usually pains in the butt. They are always complaining about something, demanding, never satisfied, controlling, and laying blame with anyone who is a willing target. They do this so you feel guilty enough or emotionally beaten down to give them what they need. If you don't, then you pay the price of judgment, criticism, sometimes rage and violence. Either version is completely self-absorbed, every moment about getting their needs met, as they truly believe the only way they can do that is from outside of themselves. I have had clients that steadfastly deny they program their actions to get and see themselves as completely selfless, giving and caring people and actually they are....but always if you dig a little deeper, you find the resentment. There is always a conditional price to be paid and that is where the buried anger comes from. You have to compromise in the giving to get, at the cost of your own nurturing. You usually find yourself always second or worse yet, last on everyone's list. You are dependent on outside attachments to make you feel loved, safe, valued, worthy and nurtured by what you do for others. That rule applies whether you are a passive or aggressive version of feeling invisible. Whether you do it silently or screaming, it is still victim energy.

The more harmonious version of the Inner Child's needs being met is: "What About Me, What About Me?" Now I know they sound as though they mean the same thing but they do not. This is where the ego gets tricky with you and tries to justify to the Inner Child it is ok to disregard and compromise your basic need of self-love, value and worthiness. In other words, how do you honestly feel about yourself? Do you like who you are, do you like what you do, do you take care of your body with respect, honor and love, do you treat others as you would like to be treated? The list goes on and on. The dark side of these needs is the closeted secrets that you hide behind, seen by others with masks of false righteousness, generosity and kindness. We are now seeing many secret closets opening with the new energy on earth. That energy of light is shining on the darkness that fear is creating very intensely now. We are seeing in the news many horrific, shameful and embarrassing details coming to light, being long hidden by religious, political and your friendly next door neighbor. The dark truths exposed will leave you with no illusions about how you really feel within. If you are hiding dark fearful secrets, you are guaranteed there is a lot of self-hatred within you that cannot exist in this new light energy. Regardless of what you have done and what secret you believe you need to hide, what only matters is how you feel about yourself and those secrets.

The statement of "What About Me?" puts how YOU feel about yourself first and then you make all your choices from that place. There is a reason when you are on an airplane and they tell you when the oxygen masks drop, to put yours on first and then the child next to you second. You must take care of yourself first

before you can be of any help to others. If you
are not functioning from a place of strength
and authenticity, you begin the dance of lying
to yourself and others about your motives. If
you live every day self-aware ("What About
Me?") and work at avoiding being self
absorbed ("It's All About Me!"), then you are
on the right track. Live in this energy and there
is no reason for dark hidden secrets as YOU are
your own guardian of the closet gate!

USING THE TOOLS YOU ARE GIFTED WITH

When you write your life script, you bring whatever tools and gifts to help complete your little adventure in this Disneyland you created. I was blessed and also knocked about in life with the gifts I came in with. As a child, I endured being touched, harassed and tricked on by the spirit realm on a daily occurrence. That spirit realm drawn to whatever bright life light I was displaying. I denied these gifts as a young adult because it was not very cool to be seeing and hearing things that you cannot touch or see, at least if you were not high on drugs at the time. There was also the issue of it completely interfering with my partying. When I finally did acknowledge them, I of course made a total fool of myself in the beginning. When all my gifts awakened, I found myself under the tutelage of many gifted but very strange and bizarre people. I guess my divine self thought I was mature enough by then to handle it with wisdom and good judgment, yeh right! My gifts fall into the categories of being a clairaudient, empathic, clairvoyant and intuitive. I have a personal aversion to saying I have psychic gifts as unfortunately that label has gotten a bad rap by all the misunderstanding of what being connected to other realms of information and energy actually means. The uninformed want to just lump us all as being the fat lady with a crystal ball and head scarf, (sorry my own issue). Most all the females in my family line have intuitive gifts to some degree or another. I also seem to be able to connect and decipher the energetic and emotional patterns that make up our soul's journey. I hear information from guides, the angelic realm, and the divine self. I can easily get behind the ego's mask and tune in on the true authentic self who wrote the script for your journey. It is pretty much impossible to con or lie to me about how you actually feel about yourself or a situation because of these gifts. I can tell you without reservation, that it did not make me a very popular or a well liked child growing up. Adults really do NOT like children seeing all their bullshit and me having a gregarious personality, I told them what I knew about everything! Pretty cheeky for a kid but also pretty dumb!

I will also admit to having some very radical out there notions you might call radical about what we are actually here doing in this life. I believe the life we are living does not have any solid outcome but is something like a virtual reality game. It is a very real experience and definitely not an illusion but you are the game programmer. The soul is having this grand experience and the divine self plays the role in this Disneyland event as the watcher, teacher and guide. It all matters on some level but in the end, it is just your soul experiencing a learning journey, nothing more. We have this sense of separation from our divine self or God self because we believe this is a solid experience and counts for everything. Most of us believe that life is all about what we are experiencing from out there. We pray TO a God and we are going TO a heaven or TO a hell. If we are good here then something meaningful will happen after this life based on the judgment of some divine being that is more than YOU. My reality is it is all US; we are doing the creating, the manifesting and the experiencing by our own choice as One and the same as we call God. You make this life work by keeping a connection to the watcher of this virtual reality game, your divine self who guides you through this journey. Once you begin to understand that you are making this up as you go along based on your emotional beliefs and you are just a character in a play, you can then make all the judgments go away. The judgments that look and sound like, is this wrong, is this right, what if, and all the should haves, would haves and could haves?

Of course, the end game is completely irrelevant! The only thing that really counts is who you perceive that you are and from what place are you making your choices. The divine self's point of view is you wrote the script and if you do not like how it is unfolding, then rewrite it! What most people do not understand is they absolutely have that kind of power with their life. In biblical terms, God supposedly gave us free will or free choice, meaning you are the writer of your own play here. If you believe that you are separated from God, that God is OUT THERE somewhere in the heavens where you are not, then you do not understand the kind of power you have over your life. The God self is within you, you being a small spark of that divine intelligence, co-creating this magnificent experience called life. That real power in your life is manifesting the attitude and gratitude you focus on when you meet life's challenges. Are you always complaining and bitching about what is NOT working in your life or are you co-creating in power to change things to the better just by your energy, thoughts and behavior? What you focus and put your energy on and the choices made is the free will that creates your life experience as an incredible Disneyland ride or a nightmare. It is truly and entirely up to you.

No one is making any of those choices for you, but YOU!

WHO IS REALLY IN CHARGE OF YOUR LIFE?

When I had my therapy practice, I did a combined program of emotional addiction, holistic and intuitive counseling. I used my abilities to see behind the ego's mask of defenses. I have the gift to see the real you, your true journey and the script you are trying to unfold for yourself. I had created an emotional and spiritual healing self-hypnosis program called Empowered Thinking that you slept with at night. It was a successful program and was definitely the foundation for me to discover the concept of Soul Windows. I am also a licensed minister, certified healer and few other blah, blah titles. I acquired a few licenses and certifications in different modalities mostly due to having a child's curiosity about everything. When presented with an opportunity to learn something new that would help me grow spiritually and energetically, I would give it a try. I believe it was that curiosity more than a desire to be a healer or whatever label that is, that finally made me realize I had a lot of information and skills to help people learn how to empower themselves. It was also a journey filled with a big ego at times. It seems if you take the path as a healer or spiritual teacher of any sort, you inevitably stumble over your own ego. You can get to thinking you are someone pretty special and awesome when you discover those gifts and start using them successfully.

When I started my emotional addiction counseling practice, I would make customized tapes for each client and kept notes of their issues on index cards. All their fears, insecurities, hopes and dreams that were wrapped around the problems they came to see me for ended up on a 4 x 6 card. After several years of doing these customized tapes, I had one of THOSE conversations with myself. I realized I had to find an easier way to give each of my clients a hypnosis program. The problem was to figure out how to make tapes that would work without all the extra effort involved. I am a firm believer if there is an easier way to accomplish an end to a project, show me. As I listened to clients all say the same things over and over again, and pretty much the same things as everyone else regardless of age, gender, marital status and life situations, it all came down to one desire….all about being loved and feeling good about you. You can call it many things and put many faces on it but love and self worth is what everyone wanted in life. Everything that is done, said, reacted to, felt and manifested is created to experience self-love and worth. You then make a choice of what your definitions of love and worth are. I have shocked many clients by saying even the seemingly most evil person and deeds have some foundation of love. I used Hitler as an example of that horrendous, distorted love. In all the pain and horrific deeds he brought about to millions, in his demented mind he believed he was purging his beloved Germany of undesirable people. He made every decision based on his love for his homeland Germany. He wanted Germany to exist in his definition of what love of his country looked like. That theory also applies to abusive relationships. Love is the only experience you are meant to have in this existence in whatever form shows up, the lack of it is everything else.

I decided to sort out all my index cards by issues, thinking I would come up with some form of a catalogue I could standardize the hypnosis tapes. Maybe even write a book about my experiences of finding the answers for clients, now how hilarious is that! By this time, I was fairly sure I had something that worked from several years of using the program. Clients were making spectacular changes in their self-esteem, confidence, feeling happier with themselves and their lives. I should make note that before I started using this program on clients, I used it myself for more than a year and personally knew it worked.

What I discovered when breaking down the index cards, it all came down to just four important categories in life. Of course, each in one's own definition but still the same. Regardless of what tribe they came from, their age, or marital status, everyone wanted to feel love and good about themselves. From the information I catalogued, the Empowered Thinking Hypnosis Program came about based on four categories:

I am Important - Mind
Unconditional Love - Heart
Forgiveness - Spirit
Health - Body

These are the basic core wants of everyone: they want to feel valued and unconditionally loved without having to compromise their self-respect or self-love. They want to be able to forgive themselves for allowing the hurtful things that happened to them and be able to forgive the perpetrators of those hurtful things. All forgiveness happens when judgment is released of the could haves, should haves or would haves we inflict upon ourselves. The last is everyone wants to be healthy. Without your health, everything else in life seems insignificant. If balanced in the first three, good health is pretty much a given byproduct just by being in harmony with your body. I created the Empowered Thinking program, keeping it simple and down to basics, on the emotional level of the Inner Child. I used this program with clients for several years with the emotional addiction and intuitive counseling. The combination helped clients to understand their core issues by changing their thinking on a sub-conscious level and the emotional responses would change their behavior. It was and still is a very effective program. I only recommend the program now when someone is in health crisis, extreme fear or emotional abandonment as the new energy on earth has changed so drastically. Most spiritual students now need more than basics; they want to understand where their power is coming from. I also later switched the sequence of the Empowered Thinking CD program, making Unconditional Love the first foundation listened to instead of I am Important. With the new ascension and cleansing vibrations on earth, much self-hatred and the lack of loving energy in general is now being addressed by everyone. No more burying, hiding or ignoring of secret issues is allowed.

How Change Begins In Our Subconscious Beliefs

Empowered Thinking For The Inner Child

Unconditional Love

The first and most important emotional foundation is Unconditional Love. This is the definition of feeling loved without having to do anything, be anything or compromise feeling good about you. In my estimation, I would say that 99.9% of most everyone you know is clueless about what that would feel and look like. The closest thing that I could describe it would be what some call the rapture or the Oneness where you are completely detached from the good opinion of others, totally disconnected to the outcome of any situation and 100% connected to the divine source. Trying to explain what unconditional love would feel and look like to someone who has never experienced it would be similar to explaining Godiva chocolate to someone who has never tasted chocolate of any kind.

Chocolate is just a chocolate word until they have tasted and experienced a version of chocolate to be able to make a comparison of the two. Unconditional love is fearless in quality and a knowing that comes from the heart. A knowing that you deserve to be loved, just because you are you, regardless of what that may look like to others. NO conditions attached! You do not have to be, do, get, have or compromise anything in expectation of being loved in a kind, caring, respectful and compassionate nature. You are exquisite in your humanity not in spite of your flaws but because of your wonderful flaws. Perfection is filled with judgment of self and others and not something that is attainable in this experience called life. Humanity exists in rules made by the ego based on everything that will make us happy is out there. To the ego, getting love is a begging, manipulative or controlling game that will always compromise how you feel about yourself participating. For example, my father will love me if I marry a rich man, have career success and make him proud. My mother will approve of me if I behave and act like her, do not shame or embarrass her. The lists are endless. In partnerships, you attract someone with the same belief foundations and issues that you have. The balance being that one is aggressive and one is passive in how they participate with those issues.

I had a client lose her challenge to cancer who was a classic case of passive conditional love designed by the ego to get her needs met. She was the giving mother who did everything for her children, family, friends, husband and always leaving herself last on the list because she believed her value only came from giving. She must give first in order to even have half a chance of getting some of her needs met. It is a bargain designed by the ego, only allowing her to feel loved when she is meeting others emotional needs first. She was taught that definition of love as a child and though it looked like unconditional love, in reality it was always living with the rules of having to give to get. The ego will even sacrifice your body if it believes it can make a last ditch effort to receive unconditional love. Your ego will convince the Inner Child of this and will take you to your deathbed and then all of a sudden the soul realizes the cost of this conditional love, "Oh shit, I can't turn this around now!" There is a point the body cannot heal itself when the soul's life force cocoon has unraveled too far and you are now heading home.

This client created cancer in her life to set up a situation to justify being able to receive love without any guilt but she still was not able to nurture herself to get well. The moment she started feeling just a little better, she was doing this for that person and errands for her grown kids. When she finally got so bad needing daily assistance and her children expressed resentment on having to give up their time to attend to her needs, she passed very quickly after that. She became aware in that moment she still could not control how love came to her no matter what she did. She never understood that getting better was just for her, not just to get well so she could continue to be this wonderful saintly mother or friend. Her definition of love was everybody else came first. She was the giver, the helper, the fixer, the one everyone turned to for help. She needed the feeling of being the loving selfless martyr. That was how she got her conditional love fix. She was mourned by hundreds when she passed and there were many stories of how she was always there for them in their times of need. When she needed to give to herself that same loving energy she gave so freely to everyone else, it was a completely, foreign concept to her and caused her to ultimately lose the physical and emotional force to sustain a reason to stay here.

The two things that we do physically and spiritually alone on our life journey are dis-ease and dying. Whether we choose to include our divine self in the challenge is the drawing card as to whether you will survive. No matter what is going on out there, you are the only one who can make the decision on getting well or calling game over and going home. It makes no difference how wealthy you are, how famous you are, how powerful you are or how loved you are, no one can do it for you. You cannot pay someone, your loved ones cannot take your place and you cannot bully nor beg it away. You must totally embrace the concept of being in love with you in order to heal your body and heart. This is a journey you must take connected to the One source, the divine spark of a divine creator. You must learn to love who you are through the divine self. I always say, you must see yourself through God's eyes, loving yourself unconditionally and without judgment. Knowing you are awesome, regardless!

When you are in ego, it impossible to see beyond your immediate needs and getting them met. You cannot gauge what you are really giving up in order to have those needs met at that moment. The ego is suspicious at best and malicious most of the time, so when you are in ego all rules will be manipulated. The gloves are off and fear is what rules the moment. When you are giving to get, it may seem like it is a selfless act but it is really being willing to sacrifice your body, your life, your respect, your self esteem to get YOUR needs met. Ego is totally and completely all about YOU getting your needs met at any cost! When you are in authentic energy of self love connected to the Divine source, then you can gauge every situation by asking a simple question, "What value am I really getting out of this?" and stay completely focused on your own journey. The difference between the first statement of "It's All About Me!" is totally self absorbed and attached to the outcome connected to everything outside of yourself. The second statement of "What About Me?" is grounded in the energy of "I am going to do what is best for me in strength and compassion, regardless of outside circumstances". Many people call that selfish but the bottom line is if you do not value you, no one else is going value you either. Your life will always reflect back your own value system in the manner of how you are treated, respected and loved. When centered in the authenticity of divine self, you are willing to honestly ask what your real needs are and take complete responsibility for getting them met without compromise.

Ego's greatest tool to keep you from doing that and THE biggest manipulative tool out there is GUILT! The moment you begin to place yourself first in any situation, that little pang in your stomach creeps up and you begin to doubt. Of course, if you don't create it yourself, everyone within 100 miles of you will take up the slack and pile all the guilt on you based on their needs not being met. The challenge for you usually comes in the question of: "How could you say no to me when I am in need?" "How could you be so selfish and place yourself first?" You might think if you say no, there is a good possibility they will not love you anymore and be there for you. If you have never asked anyone for anything directly, they will probably not be aware that you need something anyway. When that chatter begins from the ego, you have to learn to how to stomp your foot and tell the ego to *SHUT UP!!* After awhile, it will start feeling good knowing you have that kind of power. You will be able to discern when being manipulated by ego through guilt by how you would feel if you give in or give up because of someone else's need. This is where bravery can come in handy facing down that guilt trip. The ego loves to keep you in pain and guilt and your divine self just wants you to feel good, loved and to have a good time while you are in this life experience.

I Am Important!

The second foundation to build on is I Am Important, which is feeling valued and worthy. The issue is always the same, where DO you get your value and worth from? Is it outside of yourself: depending on marital status, money, job, appearance, clothes, fame or family to say you have worth and value? The second part of that equation is what ARE your definitions of value and worth? In other words, you must get your priorities straight. This script for the program drove home the point that your value and worth comes from that you are breathing! You are here having a soul experience and as far as your divine self sees it, just doing that is an awesome adventure! Your divine self gets to experience this life through you. That is what Oneness is about, understanding there is no separation between the awesome God Self that resides within you and the character that is experiencing your life. It is One and the same but most of us view our life based on experiences and material things that have no value when we spiritually go home. If for some reason, you made the decision to sit in a field naked for the rest of your life, Ooooming everyday until dusk, your divine self would think that was pretty cool if YOU thought it was wonderful too! The crumbling foundations of your value and worth are built on beliefs given to you growing up. You have to find what is authentic for YOU and how YOU feel about your own worth and value. That is ALL that counts, <u>ALL</u> that counts! Ooooming in a field naked, being a rock star, housewife or president is all the same to the divine self as long as you are happy and joyful doing it. Not for any underlying reasons or beliefs of what you have to be, to do or have in order to be of value and worth in other's eyes. Doing anything for the approval of others is worthless to your soul's growth. The imbalance in your worth comes from the belief you are missing something that would make you special if you had a lot of money, were married, have the incredible career, famous for something or have your parents approval, just pick your poison as they say. Once you can define what your value and self worth is based on, then you can honestly begin to look at your feelings if you were not that, did not have that something or someone or the "IT" would be missing from your life. It would most likely be feelings of less than, fearful, angry, judgmental, blaming but mostly fearful.

FORGIVENESS

The third emotional foundation is Forgiveness, which encompasses forgiveness of self first, then allows forgiveness of others. The rule for personal healing, is you must experience it yourself in order to be able to understand and share it with others. I gave an affirmation to many clients who were big into the blame game to help them move out of being unforgiving of people or situations from the past. It goes something like this: "I forgive myself for believing the lie that I am worthless and have no value and for nothing I ever did". I tell them to try not to think on it too hard and just say it for several weeks. Most people's reaction to it is..."huh, I don't feel that way about myself?" People are always so sure that contentment and peace will come after they have forgiven someone else. They do not realize they are actually pissed at themselves for allowing whatever. We all have something that our Inner Child has not forgiven us for that we had to give up, made to do, could not make happen or could not stop. When you have been abused in any form, never got the answers to why you were not loved the way you knew you deserved or abandoned to emotionally or physically fend for yourself, the Inner Child will always assume the responsibility unless given other answers. The list is long and brutal. If you have ever dealt with a four year old having a temper tantrum, you know the only way to satisfy that emotional fit is to replace it with something loving and filled with trust. Forgiveness of self comes from finally realizing you do not have to take the responsibility for someone else's pain, bad treatment of you or the inability to love you as you deserved. You must place the responsibility where it needs to go, on the choices they made about you. Accepting that it was not about what you were or what you were not. The ego in it's neediness to find importance for it's existence is willing to make even those events special for you by making you believe that you had that kind of power to do something about those hurts when you were young. You have to unload that burden first. You were a little kid, for God's sake! What the hell did you know about being responsible for an adult's choices? You thought your parents and all the adults in your life knew everything.

By the time a client reached the Forgiveness CD, the process was like peeling an onion. After a few layers of self-realization, it started getting pretty intense when you finally reach the layer I called, "poking the sleeping bear". It is your divine self's tool to bring up the old buried emotions keeping you from feeling empowered, balanced, content and just basically being joyful in this life journey. Oh and of course, do what you intended to do here, unload the burdens of ego that keep you from divine Oneness. You will know when your divine self has taken the drivers seat in your life when you have over the top reactions or you hear yourself saying those famous words of, "Wow! didn't see that coming!" It means to catch you unawares so buried emotions can come roaring up and not give you time to create defenses from the ego. Emotions are the tools of the divine self to let you know something is not quite right in your life or on the upside when you have brought things into balance. When you are fearful, angry, resentful, insecure, hateful or jealous, it is your divine self's way of giving you a heads up that something needs addressed on your journey and the time is now. If you are in a situation when things seem to be going well and then all of a sudden you get your buttons pushed from out of nowhere, do not look at it as a bad thing. It gives you the opportunity to ask yourself why you felt that way, what made you act that way and how did you just give your power away to someone by word or action. That is called poking the sleeping bear, sometimes it is only a nudge and growl and then sometimes it becomes a full on attack of emotional or physical challenging proportions. A good gauge of knowing you have been poked, is the feeling of being blindsided by someone's comment or action, an unexpected disappointment or a situation that creates unreasonable fear or anger. If you can honestly say, "Wow, I did not see that coming!" you can be guaranteed your divine self has made a life journey decision for you to speed up the process or to get one going.

HEALTH

On the subject of good health, it is simply a given when the first three foundations are addressed. We then have the ability to experience a natural harmonious balanced body. The vehicle that houses your soul throughout this life journey is designed by you to experience the lessons as needed. The body is meant to be in perfect health, functioning effortlessly. Now I know the first thing that pops up in everyone's mind is what about deformities and handicaps from birth. The obvious when following the rules that you wrote the script is the soul desired that experience to be in a body with limitations. It does not necessarily mean the lesson is for the soul who inhabits the handicapped body, it may be a lesson for the parents and family involved. Once again, it comes down to how you emotionally deal with the challenges you wrote in your life script. Are you going to feel sorry for yourself because you are thinking maybe God has punished you for something by not having a perfect child or being born that way yourself? The other choice is praying for the inner strength to understand and overcome the challenge everyday with love, hope and compassion for everyone involved. You can always make it a better situation by how you emotionally handle it. You know the cute saying: you have a choice of making chicken soup or chicken shit out of what happens in your life.

Your body is an intelligence that thinks for itself, responds and reacts to everything you put into it and do to it. You do not consciously make your lungs work, your heart beat, digest your food or put your body into motion. Everything from the moment of your first breath is buried within your bones, muscles and organs from all energetic substances, thoughts and emotions. The body designed in perfection, will perform all the necessary functions that are needed to sustain this physical existence. What you put into the body creates a support system or forces the body to compensate to survive at all costs. I am not just talking about unhealthy food, drugs, alcohol or (what mystery meat is actually is in this?)... fast food. All negative emotions and thoughts can have an even more deteriorating effect on the body than physical substances. Those negative thoughts and emotions will push us into comfort food, drug addictions and pharmaceutical dependency.

Your body naturally functions on a level of survival at all cost, meaning it will do what it needs in to order to continue its existence and finish the intended life journey. That is why most medical diagnosis based on immediate symptoms, usually create more problems than they fix. Your body in survival mode when facing illness and dis-ease, will take life sustaining energy from a healthy organ to help a part of your body that is in distress. You must not look for someone to rescue you from the responsibilities of taking care of your own body and life. Choosing to feel entitled to do what you want to your body because of whatever excuse you can come up with always catches up with you. Everyday you should try to maintain a holistic approach of "cleaning out toxins from the body, building up the immune system (herbs and supplements) and heal and change belief foundations of loving self. Also on a daily basis, maintaining a healthy environment for the body with exercise, as much organic food you can get, as little processed food as possible and good pure, unprocessed water.

When dealing with illness, you must make choices based on your faith and convictions of what you believe will work for you. It makes no difference if you choose traditional treatment and then take the path of healing and strengthening your body from the aftermath of medical procedures or only choose the path of alternative and natural treatment. Believing you are the one healing your body is the only thing that matters, regardless of the results. That belief should be one of joyous and fearless expectation of the right outcome for you, whatever that may be. You must also work at fearlessly and lovingly embracing life to the fullest and counting every day as a precious gift and not look at your body as though it has betrayed you in some way. The hardest idea that clients had accepting when facing life threatening dis-ease, was learning how to love the dis-ease that was ravaging their body. It is a part of who they are, maybe not the great part but still a creation of their own imbalance. If you hate any part of what you are, that hated part will die within you. Your body was designed to be filled with loving energy, anything else contaminates your body vehicle and stops you from being in optimal health. I truly believe the only true control we have over our bodies is the acceptance and responsibility of those powerful choices. If we recognize how truly empowered we are in partnership with this awesome higher power and healing intelligence that shares this existence within us, we can then honor our bodies and our lives with those empowered choices. We can be in gratitude and awe of our simple everyday health choices, knowing they have the potential of committing us to the fearless responsibility for the outcome of our health and our happiness. Forgiveness and unconditional loving acceptance of self, is the only true healing there is for dis-ease. My prayer of choice was asking for assistance from all the Christ Light Powers That Be, to transform any negative thoughts, beliefs, negative karma, out of balance life imprints or genetic coding that was contributing to ill health or love of self. That prayer works for any challenge you may be facing in your life, by the way. I found the body when experiencing fearful emotions, a little hesitant with the idea of "releasing the imbalance to the light and love of God". Your body vehicle was designed to be filled with God Sparkle and love light. All energetic contained space must be filled with something, whether negative or positive. We cannot exist with an empty nothingness within our existence. Transformation versus releasing, leaves a nothing space that causes energetic fear and mistrust in the psyche. Transforming negative energies to positive God light energies is much more comforting to the Inner Child and the physical makeup of the your body vehicle. At least, that has been my experience.

I would get asked many times by clients due to my own health history, about trying new wellness products with high expectations of it working and taking care of their "dis-ease or illness". It is certainly an excellent starting place for getting healthy. Your belief foundation when using any of those wonderful "miracle" nutritional products create positive flow in the body and opens the cell channels to release dis-ease, toxins and embrace healing nutrients. The product will imprint its energy on your life force and then your body decides whether it is for you or not, like matching up a DNA search. Either it likes it, needs it or it does not. Your body always makes the choice as to whether this product is going to work for you. Bottom line is…there are NO wellness products out there that will miraculously heal you overnight! But, sometimes there are healing miracles that do happen when a supplement or treatment imprints the body under the right circumstances. A miracle is just a shift in perception and energy. That is exactly what your body will decide to do, shift into wellness when the right product is introduced into your system. The so-called miracle products work on some people for their illness and not on others. The best approach for staying well and dealing with a challenging health crisis is to understand and accept completely that you created it. Now you must ask for the assistance of the divine within to give you hand in helping you heal, make it bearable or live with the disability life dealt you. Another good question to ask of yourself is how does this illness or dis-ease serve you? Meaning, what is the ego getting out of this experience and what needs are being met? Dis-ease and disability is truly one of the hardest challenges to find some gratitude for in a life experience. One never really knows for sure what the soul's big picture is when it comes to challenges with our bodies or watching loved ones deal with them. Praying, meditation and stomping your foot once in awhile to ask for a little help from the divine are a few examples of what I know that works to help get you through them.

THE RULES OF MANIFESTING THE LIFE YOU WANT

I would explain co-creating on the terms of sending out a thought or intention, feeling, emotion or belief energetically and then the God Spark within captures that energy and blows life into it to manifest it into this reality. You are always the source of that intention, creating consciously or with buried sub-conscious programs. You are manifesting continuously, either with intent or from buried emotional beliefs in your sub-conscious. That is the foundation where ALL prayers are answered, which is actually true. The trick to having those prayers manifest into physical reality is in your capacity of receiving those prayers, with conditions or without. The divine self will always be available to manifest your intentions but if you are unable to receive the gift because of negative or unharmonious beliefs and emotions of unworthiness or doubt, your desires will not come about or your prayers answered in the way you are expecting. Negative talk, thinking, emotions and feelings literally create webbing around your etheric life force that will catch the intended manifested prayer and keep it from becoming a physical reality. Quite literally, your good gifts bounce off into nothingness or you receive a distorted or less than version of your desire. That is why it is so important to be aware of what you are creating every moment and every moment does count!

Your intentions are everything and with the new and powerful energy in this dimensional existence, you must be very, very careful of what you say, what you ask for and what you put out as your belief system. The energy is so high vibration now there is almost instantaneous manifesting of what you put into thought, word and actions. Everyone's karma is on a very short leash now. This is how we manifest our life journey: we think, we believe and then we put an intention into in the etheric realms of manifesting. For example, you say and think, "I really want a new red car." You think about it everyday and you put the joyful emotions behind it and send it to the divine ethereal realm. The divine aspect of yourself catches that emotional spark and blows life into it, manifesting it into physical reality for you. Now here is why the ability to receive without conditional beliefs is crucial. If the red car you are asking for is a brand new Porsche and your level of self value and worth at the time is only at a red Ford Focus, a Ford Focus is what is going to show up for you. This is where your soul shows you at what point your journey's growth is and gives you the perfect opportunity to make a free choice of expansion. You can be in wonderful gratitude for your beautiful, shiny, new Ford Focus and say, "OK, I was not quite able to manifest the Porsche yet but somehow and some way I will." Or you could have the attitude of, "This piece of crap, I wanted a red Porsche and this is what I got", thanks a lot God! I can guarantee the one who is thrilled to see their new Ford Focus show up in their driveway and have expectations of one day seeing the Porsche parked there, will. The one filled with resentment, less than, jealousy and envy will never even get close to owning one and more than likely as the years go by, will be driving that same Ford Focus until it falls apart. No prayers go unanswered; it is just the particulars of what actually shows that gets tricky. It states that particular phrase in many spiritual reference sources but if you ask most people going through a hard time in life about the absolute results of prayer, their answer would probably be no. Obviously, there is some misunderstanding on how much control we have in the receiving of our good. Since we are the one writing the script, we should be able to manifest exactly what we ask for, right? One would think so!

Here is why you seem to be not getting what you pray for or your life does not seem to be working out the way you hoped. Once again, it is in the receiving of what you are putting out mirroring back to you. The emotional energy behind a prayer request and intention is the important part of manifesting the exactness of what you are going to receive. Many times we pray and bind the universe's hands so tightly with conditions of what we want that it is impossible to get past our stipulations of how it should look. Well, sometimes your divine self has to create a backdoor method for you, meaning your good does not come to you on a straight line but directed through many other people and avenues of manifesting. We usually see the receiving of what we want only in our limited viewpoint. For example, if a woman is in an abusive relationship, she states that she does not understand why she keeps ending up with all the mean men who abuse her. She just wants to be married to a nice man who will love her, be kind to her and will not mistreat her. Explaining that the issue is not getting someone to love or marry them, that is the easy part. The hard part is getting someone who will honor and respect them, since that is an unknown emotional concept. The reason they are not attracted to that nice guy is their definition of love is something different. What they attract to themselves is what they believe love feels like, nothing more, nothing less. Once they change their definition of love, the abusive men will stop being attracted into their energy field. They will literally become invisible to partners who are looking to control someone through violence and fear. Like attracts like and a woman who allows an abusive man into her life is just as guilty of abuse as the partner she shares the experience with. The only difference is she allows abuse under the guise that someone else is doing it to her. That is what you call passive aggression. The reason they do not know how to change those relationships is they are incapable of receiving love on any other basis. That is what love looks like, feels like and what they are comfortable with, it may not make them happy but it is all they know. Once someone is aware they are creating the outcome of relationships from their own belief system, then you have a good start at being able to sustain a healthy relationship free of self-sabotaging drama.

Your ability to receive love is the key, what does that look and feel like to you? When you pray for a happy relationship, most people pray for someone brought TO them. Instead, pray for whatever is keeping you from receiving a happy relationship, revealed to you. Asking for assistance to have the old unhappy energy transformed from your belief system. Then hold on to your hat as they say! Of course, gratitude and more gratitude is the key factor for being content with yourself and your life. If you wanted that red Porsche and wound up with the red Ford Focus, be so in gratitude for that car in the moment. For whatever reason, receiving the red Porsche just was not in your capabilities at that time. But hey, you have the brand new red Ford Focus and it is a beauty! This is when you say:"Ok, thank you, thank you all the powers that be, for this wonderful new car that I now have in front of me and I know without a doubt that somehow, some way that new red Porsche is going to show up in my life! Then every time you see your red Porsche on the road, instead of being resentful about not having it, point at it and say "just hold on a little while longer you beautiful sweetie, you are going to be mine soon enough!"

You have to get comfortable with the idea that sometimes your divine self is in the driver's seat giving you what you need at the moment but maybe not particularly what you wanted. The reason for this is when the life veil drops; you have just forgotten you wrote it that way in your script. Your divine self takes over the situation to show you there are gaps in your feelings of worthiness and value based on what shows up versus what you asked for. The truth is, if you desire a red Porsche then you should have one, just because. Most people immediately go into the resentment, blame, anger or feelings of failure when they ask," Where's my car?" "I asked for a red Porsche and only got a cheap red Ford Focus...damn it!" It is in the gratitude expressed in the present moment that will upgrade you to your red Porsche. Of course, what I have found in spiritual growth is when you finally reach that level of gratitude; everything else shifts and changes your value and worth system. You could possibly no longer desire the red Porsche and would rather put the money elsewhere. Your priorities may change and then you are no longer attached to the status of the red Porsche. Go figure!

ENERGETIC
PERCEPTIONS

In case you have not noticed, our day-to-day living is getting a little crazy! We are in the energies of both ascension and apocalypse, which is a vibratory acceleration of awareness and cleansing. All hidden things are now being exposed from the darkness of secrecy, being drawn out into the light of truth. That is why there are now so many instances of political and religious hypocrisy exposed. Long buried and unaddressed emotional issues are also rising to the surface. In the bigger picture of humanity, you are seeing so many instances of out of control rage, buried prejudice and violence committed by people who seemingly led quiet lives. There are severe health issues in startling numbers, planetary disruptions such as cleansing tsunamis, earthquakes and hurricanes. Humanity and the planet reflect each individual imbalance existing on her. We are in what some people would call an energetic ascension, meaning we are exposed to higher vibratory frequencies to bring about a cleansing of anything that is negatively held onto in our journey. Those energetic vibrations are moving faster and faster and every living species on this planet is affected in one way or another. The current news is filled with behavior of frustration and agitation, forcing everyone to look at the heavier and darker energies we have been carrying around possibly for lifetimes. Our bodies are also reacting to those faster vibrating energies with emotional impatience, depression, health issues, worry, fear and the mind remembering long forgotten hurts, anger and resentments. What you are is a light being, if there is anything else in your body that is not light, it is now in the light of exposure. This new energy is why you are seeing some crazy things happening as the darkness within is exposed. As the energy is moving faster on this planetary dimension, it is forcing everyone to look at what has been hiding behind the defenses of the ego.

When I counseled a client, they energetically looked like a big computer program with thousands of light threads throughout the body. These light threads weaved a picture of emotional and physical blocks. The soul imprinted a map, showing me where they were in life's journey. When I would ask questions and listen to their story, (and we all have a story) that circuitry board would light up to guide and direct me to see what was under the ego's human illusion in this life game. It really did not make any difference what your answers were as I was watching for the energetic emotional responses. What I was looking for was the emotional bridge from the ego's illusion to the authentic self. It is from these energetic light mappings I was able to see and interpret what blocks of denial, buried anger, secret fears or feelings of inadequacies that were keeping you from feeling love for yourself and feeling good about your life. For example, when I asked someone what their relationship was like with their mother and I got an answer of "well she was a little hard to please", what I saw inside was a pinball effect of emotions bouncing around from rage, control and feelings of never enough. I would gently try to make them aware it was ok to feel those buried emotions but maybe time to stop dealing with them like a child. The child, who will never figure out how to please their mother or whomever and to start learning how just please you. The impossibility of receiving unconditional love or value by that person was probably never going to happen and needed to be let go. There was always lots of resistance from the Inner Child on that one, as she is the perpetual child of someday I can make it happen or make that go away if only I do this, think this or don't do this or don't think this. Then of course, the other approach is to lie to yourself and say you don't care if you please her or anyone and become the rebellious child. You pick a defense program around four to seven years of age and run with it the rest of your life. As I would watch these energetic emotions bounce around during the interview and continuing conversation, I usually discovered most people are aware of their inharmonious feelings. They have either learned to live with them or have tried all kinds of fix it self-help on every level and believe they are making some headway with the problems. In a lot of cases this is true but after all the intellectualizing about what it is and what it isn't, I always would just bring it down to one important question for them. Asking, "Well, I know how you feel about everyone and everything else but how do you actually feel about yourself? It usually did the trick. Most of the time I got blank stares, a "what do you mean" look or just plain stuttering as they had never even considered the question before.

We had now reached the point where I could ask the hard question, "If you had a mother, father, husband or boss that has made you feel insignificant, less than, abused, without value or worth, why would you love someone like that and put up with their bad behavior?" After some interesting answers like,

"Because she is my mother, I need my job, I love them or I don't want to be alone." I would begin to narrow the path in getting them to understand that was their definition of love, value or worth. That is why they continued to accept all that drama in their life, even though it did not make them happy. They may not like it but it is all they know, like a computer program running in the background they must obey. In abusive relationships, I would ask a woman why she stayed with or kept going back to their partner and the answer usually was..."I don't know why, I just love him". "Why are earth would you love someone who would mistreat you and hurt you, why?" Have you ever asked yourself that question? The answer would be, it is the only definition of love you know and taught to you from someone else. Does that mean you have to live with that definition the rest of your life, no you do not! Time to change it!

IT'S ALL YOU!

This life journey belongs only to YOU, with you making all the decisions from that vantage point. As I mentioned before, dis-ease and dying are the two great equalizers when it comes to experiencing authenticity in your life, you make the choice to get better and live OR you do not. I got asked by clients who made the same natural healing choices as I did fifteen years ago, why it worked for me and not for them. I chose to heal myself of stage four breast cancer naturally without chemo or surgery. My answer had many possibilities but I started with telling them the first thing I did was make myself an absolute priority. I trusted my instincts and did not allow outside influences to tell me what I could or could not accomplish with my body. The bottom line was I did not allow myself to buy into the medical fear that pushes you into making drastic and brutal choices to heal. You do not look for someone or something to "heal" you. YOU are the healer of your own imbalance. You can get all the help you want but ultimately the choice remains yours. Cancer is just a fungus, albeit a very aggressive one but still just a fungus. One of the tools I used was continually focusing only on the results I wanted and giving no credibility to any dis-ease. Heck, I sometimes forgot I even had it during the process. People would come up to me in that whispery voice they use when they think they are being polite about a touchy subject and ask how <u>WAS</u> I doing? I would stand there a few seconds wondering, why the heck were they talking to me like that? Then it would dawn on me, "oh yeh, they are asking me about how the cancer is going?" I found it extremely amusing that I inevitably was the one who consoled and reassured the person I was talking too. Life, huh? It can get pretty, ridiculous sometimes.

The need to be right is what also destroys most relationships and eventually destroys any chance of being happy and content with yourself and life. It affects every arena of your life. When the need to be right is the rule in anyone's life, there is always hurt that follows. You get to express your righteousness and make your point at all cost and usually the costs are very high. You have arguments, racial inequality, religious judgment, crushing fragile hearts, ending human life, greed and malicious intent all in the energy of believing that you are the only one that is right. The ego loves it! The divine self just sighs and gently nudges you in the direction of helping you to see it really does not matter who is right and who appears to be wrong. The only thing that matters is dealing with everyone and everything in loving energy, beginning with you. I am not talking about keeping your mouth shut all the time in avoidance as that is dishonesty in the most, manipulative form. You can speak your truth and as long as you are not attached to it being accepted as being their truth and respect and honor the old saying of agreeing to disagree, then you have harmony for both parties. Or at the very least, for you.

Another insidious tool of the ego is the mastery of a good feel sorry for you episode. Sometimes it is just good to wallow around in your pity party awhile but then you must take responsibility to bring about change for the better. Here are three guidelines that can help stop the pity party.

1. Find anything to be in Gratitude for. Even the smallest blessing will help change the energy with viewing a situation as a glass ½ full versus being ½ empty.

2. Have Faith in yourself that you have what it takes somewhere within you to find your Muchness (self-confidence and self-empowerment) to get through this challenge. If you doubt you have it, ask the divine powers to help you find it!

3. Trust that you are not doing this challenge alone! You are connected and always part of an awesome divine energetic source that will help. Call it prayer, meditation or whatever! Just embrace Gratitude and have the Faith and Trust in your divine partnership for a perfect outcome! Even if you have to stomp your foot like a little kid and say, "You know, I need a little help here!" Go on and do that, it will make you feel much better!

LIVING A QUALITY RELATIONSHIP WITH YOU

In counseling clients in miserable relationships, many new clients would be a little, taken aback with my approach at their first interview session. I gave them about 5 or 10 minutes of complaining and bitching about how miserable their partnership was and then I would politely stop the blah, blah, blah with this statement, "Well I think we have heard enough about what your partner contributes to this miserable situation, how about let us look at what you are contributing". Until one got used to the counseling I did, I had to make it clear I was not there to listen to them vent for an hour. We were there for them to find out why they had created a situation in their life that needed venting and to take responsibility for it. The usual reaction was one of denial and continued blame. Eventually I could get around to asking them the important question of what they were contributing to the situation and why? After all, it is extremely difficult to create a miserable relationship all by yourself. It is also difficult to heal a relationship if someone has never heard the concept that you are creating everything in your life by your belief system and thought process. This is always a good starting point to get their thinking around the idea they must take responsibility for everything that is going on in their life, whether they are conscious of it or not. I would ask these questions: "what do you want for yourself, who do you think you are in the relationship, why do you think you are not getting what you want in life"? The moment they would go back to the dialogue of, he did, she said, he has, I steered the conversation back to them. When you are in a conflict with someone, you must stay away from the statements: "you are, you did, you have, you think, you must or didn't". Everything is then outside of yourself and the power of the outcome is placed on the person you are having a conflict with. If you keep the dialogue in, "I think, I want, I feel or I do", then you are only taking responsibility for your own contribution to the conflict. Of course, the best calming statement you can say to someone is, "what is it that you want from me or what is it that I can do for you to make this right?" It takes the steam right out of the situation and will immediately change it to a lighter energy as you have acknowledged their needs too!

Relationships can be a very good gauge to see how well you are doing in the "It's All

About Me!" or "What About Me" game. Co-dependence is based on these very rules of giving to get your needs met. All couples who make life contracts to learn from each other have an agenda. Your partner is there to teach you what you believe is missing from you and the only way to get it is from someone else. Sometimes it comes in the package of learning how to nurture you from the complete lack of it in an abusive relationship. It may come in learning the value of your own nurturing skills. As you give to others, you learn that you are allowed to give to yourself first. The best partnerships are based on both partners needing nothing from each other and loving themselves more than they love their partner or equally at best. When I first got married, I understood this lesson very clearly. I had a long history of believing I had to beg for love until I got that lesson of, "I Am All That"! I told my husband if at anytime he discovered he was not happy being with me, he was more than welcome to leave. It was not because of any feelings of betrayal or victim energy on my part. The reasoning behind that statement was I absolutely did not want anyone that did not think I was the most wonderful woman in his life. If he thought someone else could make him happier, I wanted that for him too. It had nothing to do with him not wanting me anymore but only with knowing that I deserved to have someone in my life respectful and honorable about the love I was offering. The joke between us married to an intuitive was if he ever considered straying from the marriage, I would probably know it even before he did, so why bother. Of course I always ended the conversation with, "I want you to be happy with your choice but don't let the door hit you on your butt on the way out as you can be sure someone else is happily waiting to take your place". That is what you call a "Personal Tude", knowing you are coming to the table with something fabulous! The most important part of that statement is I meant it without doubt! I am not in the least bit manipulated by my ego or Inner Child when it comes to the belief that I am loveable and without any conditions attached to it. I know that for sure and without doubt as I paid my dues long enough living the other truth in believing I had to beg for love. I put up with demeaning treatment and abusive conditions to feel loved at any cost. Then I had that awakening and slapped myself on the forehead and said out loud mind you......"What the heck was I thinking!" It was the epiphany!

I often heard from clients when they met someone new about how he was this, he was that, and gave me this and had this and that and how wonderful he made her feel. My response usually stopped their euphoria and gave them some serious thought about their Muchness and Personal Tude. I would ask them, "And what exactly wonderful are YOU bringing to the table that he would value?" I watched for the pause and look of realization that they never thought of that! That statement is the most crucial key to a relationship to stay out of the co-dependence drama. You have to know you are not with someone with only the expectations of how they are going to make you happy. Inevitably, they will fail at it because you are the only one who truly knows what happiness feels like for you. That partner can give you a temporary version of it but it is like holding your breath, sooner or later you have to breath, giving in to your own needs and desires being made a priority...and rightly so. Once again, it all comes down to how YOU feel about yourself not how others feel about you. The blame game in relationships is an amazingly powerful tool of the ego. That is why when you are in an argument with a partner or with anyone, you must keep it all about your feelings and your actions. You cannot know or assume the intentions, thoughts or feelings of anyone else. An extreme example of this is someone using violence against another person and blaming the person violated. Claiming if that person had only behaved, not said or not did something, they would not have hurt them. The perpetrator of that violence will take no responsibility for a choice made by them and them alone. Someone like that blames everything that happens in their life to outside circumstances. Violence is always a symptom of self-hatred. Anger is a powerful tool of the ego to be right at all costs and when escalated to a point of being out of control rage, is when physical violence comes into play.

Creating A Life You Like

In order to have even the slightest inclination as to whom you really are, you must start asking questions that have no attachment to anyone or anything in your life. What is it that YOU really want out of life, where would YOU really like to live, what would YOU really like have for a career, what kind of partner would YOU really be happy with, what would YOU really like to feel about your body and health, and on and on and on. I would always like to ask these questions with the beginning phrase of: "If I had a magic fairy wand and I could wave it right now and give you the perfect life, what would that look like?" The reason I did this was to get them to start thinking of the possibility of actually creating what they really wanted out of life. Letting go of the idea they must settle for circumstances they feel stuck with in the moment. The beauty of having this human experience is you get the opportunity to learn how to unconditionally love yourself, not in spite of your flaws and shortcomings but because of them. You are having a soul experience and regardless of what it may appear to be from the perspective of your tribal laws, family values, legalities and moral judgments, to the soul it is just the experience it wanted and created for you. A soul experiences a life journey to learn, feel and release the emotions that keeps us separated from Oneness.

I have a helpful guide that loves the movies, so I am constantly being given little movie snippets that gets a point across very effectively. One of my favorite movies is "Something's Got To Give" with Diane Keaton and Jack Nicholson. There is a scene where they are having dinner in Paris for her birthday and she is a little drunk. A comment is made how she cannot hold her liquor and gets intoxicated on just one drink. Her response to that comment explains exactly the point I am trying to make. Her awesome answer was, "I like that about myself!" She acknowledges their perception of her so-called flaw, makes no apologies for it and embraces the supposed flaw as part of who she is. That is what unconditional love and acceptance of self looks like when the divine is trying to guide the soul. Life is not about the soul trying for perfection, not possible! It is about the acceptance of everything and learning everything about who you really are: a spiritual being having a human experience, nothing more than that. So when you think you do stupid things, fall on your face in embarrassment and humiliation, you cry and think you have failed, become disappointed in yourself and life in general, it is just the journey. Sometimes there are points in your life you feel amazing about yourself and other times not so much. The whole point of the life journey is to learn to not be attached to what you have done but being in complete and unconditional acceptance of who is making the choices during the experience, YOU!

While I have expounded on the point that this journey only belongs to you and only you have full responsibility of it, I must also point out that you do not come alone or without assistance. You signed on for this life experience and you must have other players to help unfold the journey. The gathered group that assists you is your soul family. Souls that have shared your journey for countless lives, changing characters as need be. The one thing I found the hardest for people to absorb is the idea they choose both their parents and family for the necessary karmic and genetic coding in order to have a particular life experience. I usually got an answer anywhere from:"There is no way I would actually choose my messed up parents or "You have got to be kidding, what the hell was I thinking!" Every player in your life agrees to all the well laid out plans before incarnation. So sometimes when you have the worst relationship with family or love partner, it is the most loving soul family member who agreed to be the so called thorn in your side in order for you to be able to address strong emotions buried within you or again maybe not. One really never knows what karma is held between two people who have big issues to deal with. Only that resolution is wanted.

You would be surprised at how shocked some are when they realize they have never given any thought to who they might be if their identity was detached from everyone and everything. The bottom line in any phase of your life is what do YOU feel, what are YOU thinking and what choices are YOU going to make based on how YOU perceive yourself. It is pretty scary to some folks. I would get asked many times in counseling sessions, the one big question of..."Can you tell me what my life's purpose is?" I guess my answer was fairly disappointing compared to what they were expecting from me. Most were obviously looking for a deep spiritual and profound perspective on the big picture of life and how they fit into that scenario? I could give a general guide book answer to what they wanted to accomplish on their journey but the bottom line of anyone's life purpose is to know love in every conceivable form, not separated from anyone or anything in that search for Oneness. How you play that out on your life journey is your own fingerprint. My belief is when we surrender our physical form and go home, whatever that may be, your accumulation of wealth, success, accomplishments, family, how much you were loved or hated, respected or revered means very little or nothing. The end game is entirely about how YOU feel about how you lived your life. My rule of thumb has always been if you cannot take it with you, it is worthless to your spiritual journey. I think the only two questions you will be asked upon arriving home are, "How were you of service to your spiritual family and how do you love yourself?" That is what you will take with you from one incarnation to the next. The real purpose of your life is being of service in whatever form that comes for you and learning to love and accept yourself unconditionally as Oneness. Important service can come in the form of making someone smile in the grocery line, helping an elderly person with packages and all the way up to total self-sacrifice for a cause. It is your script to write. Lifting someone's energy up and sharing the light of hope, that is what service is. If you can accomplish a version of that everyday of your life, then you have the big picture of what life is all about! Live your life everyday, patting yourself on the back at the awesome adventure you have created. There are many different versions of you existing in many dimensions but only one God Spark that is alive within you, Oneness. That is what Oneness is: being part of that life spark of a loving divine intelligence that you reflect in every word, action or thought.

EPILOGUE

Traveling The Good Journey

In my own life journey of sharing metaphysical, holistic, emotional addiction and spiritual counseling, I evolved into many phases, offering help on a multitude of levels through the years. Some I was good at and some just so, so. Some I found I loved and as it turned out, I was very good at those gifts. They were the gifts I stayed with and developed. I discovered through much trial and error that my best ability was the desire to help people learn how to empower themselves by understanding and accepting they were co-creating their life with the divine Oneness within. In charge of whatever outcome their beliefs took them to. To help them see how absolutely, awesomely, flipping, fantabulous they are! That is what I would consider my path of service. I hope in some small way this book has also helped you see the divine self that shines through you. Calling to task all the B.S. the ego tries to make you believe that you are not All That! Bravo!

Namaste
Susan Z Rich
www.szrwhitewings.com

www.ingramcontent.com/pod-product-compliance
Lightning Source LLC
Chambersburg PA
CBHW020434290526
45785CB00002B/836